One Health for Veterinary Nurses and Technicians: An Introduction

One Health for Veterinary Nurses and Technicians: An Introduction

Edited by

Rebecca Jones
Langford Vets, Bristol, UK

and

Andrea Jeffery
University of Bristol, UK

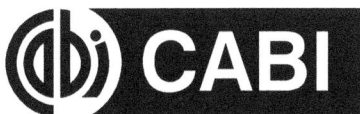

CABI

CABI is a trading name of CAB International

CABI
Nosworthy Way
Wallingford
Oxfordshire OX10 8DE
UK

CABI
200 Portland Street
Boston
MA 02114
USA

Tel: +44 (0)1491 832111
E-mail: info@cabi.org
Website: www.cabi.org

Tel: +1 (617)682-9015
E-mail: cabi-nao@cabi.org

A catalogue record for this book is available from the British Library, London, UK.

ISBN-13: 9781789249453 (paperback)
        9781789249460 (ePDF)
        9781789249477 (ePub)

DOI: 10.1079/9781789249477.0000

Commissioning Editor: Alexandra Lainsbury
Editorial Assistant: Lauren Davies
Production Editor: Shankari Wilford

Typeset by SPi, Pondicherry, India

Contents

Contributors

Helen Ballantyne MSc PGDip BSc RVN
NHS, Cambridge, UK
Email: helen_ballantyne@yahoo.com

Emi Barker BSc BVSc PhD DipECVIM-CA
Langford Vets, University of Bristol, Bristol, UK
Email: Emi.barker@bristol.ac.uk

Paula Boyden BVetMed MRCVS
The Links Group
Email: Paula.Boyden@dogstrust.org.uk

Hayley Burdge DipAVN(Surg) VTS(Surg) RVN
Langford Vets, Bristol, UK
Email: H.J.Kilbane@bristol.ac.uk

Kirsty Cavill BSc(Hons) RVN
Paws Canine Myotherapy Care, The Vet Connection
Email: pawsmyotherapycare@gmail.com

Marta Costa DVM MSc FRC Path. DipECVP MRCVS EBVS
Bristol Veterinary School, University of Bristol, UK
Email: 4mtcosta@gmail.com

Carla Finzel RVN
District Veterinary Nurse, founder of the DVN Hub
Email: carla@dvnhub.com

Jo Hockenhull BSc MSc PhD
University of Bristol, Bristol, UK
Email: Jo.hockenhull@bristol.ac.uk

Andrea Jeffery Ed.D MSc FHEA DipAVN(Surg) Cert Ed RVN
Bristol Veterinary School, University of Bristol, UK
Email: Andrea.Jeffery@bristol.ac.uk

Rebecca Jones DipAVN(Surg) RVN
Langford Vets, Bristol, UK
Email: Becky.Jones@bristol.ac.uk

Nicola Lakeman MSc BSc(Hons) RVN CertSAN VTS(Nutrition)
IVC Evidensia, Bristol, UK
Email: Lakeman.nicola@gmail.com

Robyn Lowe FdSc DipAVN(small animal) DipHE CVN RVN
Vets 4 Pets, Wigan, UK
Email: robynlowervn@gmail.com

Ellie West CertVA DipECVAA PIEMA MRCVS
Davies Veterinary Specialists, Hitchin, UK and Linnaeus
Email: ellie.west@vetspecialists.co.uk

Introduction

Rebecca Jones[1]* and Andrea Jeffery[2]
[1]*Langford Vets, Bristol, UK;* [2]*University of Bristol, UK*

One Health, at its most basic level, is the recognition of the connections between humans, animals and the environment. This recognition is not new; throughout history there have been acknowledgments, including those by the Greek physician, Hippocrates, who recognized the interdependence of public health and a clean environment and others such as Dr Rudolph Virchow (19th century) and Dr Calvin Schwabe (20th century), who respectively first coined the terms 'zoonosis' and 'one medicine' (Evans and Leighton, 2014; Capua and Cattoli, 2018). However, it was in the early 21st century, as a response to the emerging zoonotic diseases, notably severe acute respiratory syndrome (SARS) and avian influenza H5N1, with the potential to cause pandemic outbreaks and international crises, that prompted the global recognition of the need for greater transdisciplinary collaboration (Gibbs, 2014; Destoumieux-Garzon *et al.*, 2018). The risks of these pandemics highlighted the increasing globalization of health risks and the role of the human–animal–environment interface in the evolution and continued emergence of zoonotic disease (Destoumieux-Garzon *et al.*, 2018). Other global issues of concern, including the development of other multifactorial and chronic diseases, antimicrobial resistance, food safety and security and the impacts of environmental change, have further contributed to the call for an integrated, transdisciplinary approach (Evans and Leighton, 2014; Destoumieux-Garzon *et al.*, 2018).

The publication of the Manhattan Principles on 'One World, One Health', following a symposium hosted by the Wildlife Conservation Society in 2004, formed the basis for the One Health concept of today (Cook *et al.*, 2004; Evans and Leighton, 2014). These principles listed 12 recommendations for establishing a more holistic approach to combating health threats in humans and animals and maintaining ecosystem integrity. This was followed by a tripartite agreement (a legal agreement between three parties) between the World Health Organization (WHO), the World Organization for Animal Health (OIE, formerly Office International des Epizooties) and the Food and Agriculture

*Email: Becky.Jones@bristol.ac.uk

© CAB International 2023. *One Health for Veterinary Nurses and Technicians*
(eds R. Jones and A. Jeffery)
DOI: 10.1079/9781789249477.0001

Organization of the United Nations (FAO), with a commitment to addressing risks at the human–animal–environment interface (FAO/OIE/WHO, 2010). They expanded the scope of this collaboration in 2017 with the publication of *The Tripartite's Commitment* (FAO/OIE/WHO, 2017). Since then, there have been an ever-increasing number of organizations evolving the concept of One Health, but until recently there was no universally accepted definition of One Health (Evans and Leighton, 2014).

The COVID-19 pandemic once again emphasized the need for a One Health approach and in response to this need, a One Health High-Level Expert Panel (OHHLEP) was created in 2021, expanding the original Tripartite group to include the United Nations Environment Programme (UNEP). One of the key products from their first annual report was a comprehensive definition of One Health, with the objective of developing a common language and understanding around this concept (OHHLEP, 2021). This definition is shared in Box 1.1.

It is perhaps not surprising that obtaining an agreed definition for One Health has been so elusive; the very concept of One Health means that it is dynamic and continuously evolving as new knowledge is acquired (Capua and Cattoli, 2018). Along with this, the issues faced are complex and, without the right voices at the table, proposed solutions can create other issues, so there is recognition for the inclusion of a wider range of disciplines; for example, social sciences play a major role in the issues faced under One Health (Evans and Leighton, 2014; Destoumieux-Garzon *et al.*, 2018). One Health is often depicted as three overlapping circles (Venn diagram), representing humans, animals and the environment in equal balance (Fig. 1.1). However, there can still be insufficient consideration given to all components and a major barrier to successful implementation of One Health remains the lack of communication between different disciplines, including human and veterinary medicine and other disciplines such as environmental, ecological and evolutionary sciences (Destoumieux-Garzon *et al.*, 2018).

Additionally, for One Health to become fully integrated as an approach, it cannot just exist at a global or national level; the issues faced are just as relevant at a local, community level too. The editors of this book believe that

---

Box 1.1. The One Health High-Level Expert Panel (OHHLEP) definition of One Health

One Health is an integrated, unifying approach that aims to sustainably balance and optimize the health of people, animals and ecosystems. It recognizes the health of humans, domestic and wild animals, plants, and the wider environment (including ecosystems) are closely linked and inter-dependent. The approach mobilizes multiple sectors, disciplines and communities at varying levels of society to work together to foster wellbeing and tackle threats to health and ecosystems, while addressing the collective need for clean water, energy and air, safe and nutritious food, taking action on climate change, and contributing to sustainable development.

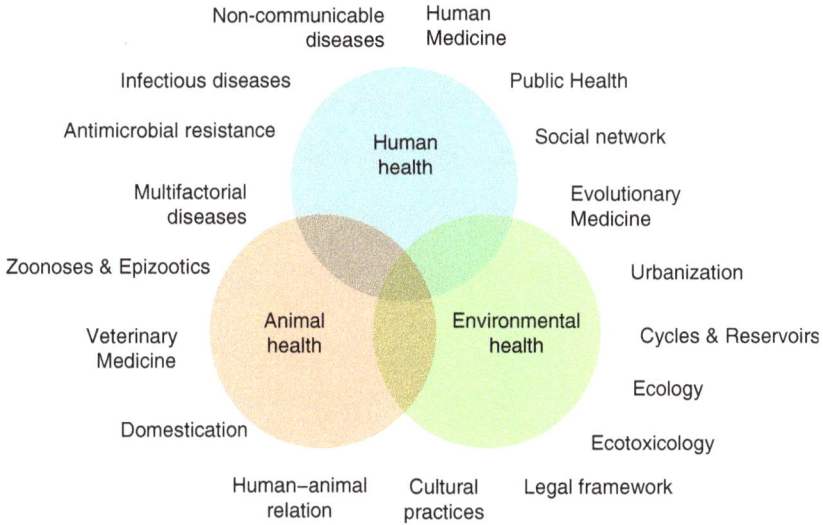

Fig. 1.1. The One Health Triad (Venn Diagram). (Attributed to Destoumieux-Garzon *et al.*, 2018; available for use under CC BY 4.0.)

this is where the veterinary nursing profession could have the most impact. As veterinary nurses, we take responsibility for the health and wellbeing of our patients and we understand that doing this effectively requires consideration of the owner too, recognizing the importance of the human–animal bond. There is also a growing public awareness of the strength of the human–animal bond, with animals often now viewed as family members and the role of assistance and therapy animals continuously evolving. Veterinary nurses have a key role to play in educating and supporting owners and caregivers by facilitating a human–animal bond that is truly mutually beneficial for both the human and the animal. There is also a need to expand our remit to include the wider community that we, our patients and their owners live within, and to recognize that this community is inclusive of all living things within it.

The COVID-19 pandemic served to raise public awareness of issues such as wildlife–human interactions, emerging infectious disease risks and the positive impact that reduced human activity could have on the environment. However, it was also a time of great uncertainty. Worldwide, people at all levels, from political leaders to members of the public, were required to navigate their way through the unknown (Nelson *et al.*, 2020). The global online platform bombarded the world with information, often from unreliable sources, including where the virus originated from, the role that companion animals had in spreading the virus and controversial opinions regarding vaccinations, heightening an already complex and anxiety-inducing situation (Nelson *et al.*, 2020). The problem of misinformation is not limited to the COVID-19 pandemic and, as healthcare professionals, we are also not immune to its effects. By appropriately educating ourselves on the issues of One Health, we can become trusted and reliable sources of information for others. It is important to note here that 'appropriate education' means seeking to understand the issues through all viewpoints, not just the ones that most closely align with our own; this is a key component of the One Health concept. With this in mind, veterinary nurses have a great opportunity to join, or even start, the transdisciplinary discussions and collaborations around One Health, having a unique viewpoint and skillset of their own to bring to the table. The chapters that follow demonstrate how One Health can, and should, become a continuous thread woven through our everyday work and lives as veterinary nurses.

It feels quite apt to end this chapter with a quote commonly attributed to the 18th century writer and poet, Samuel Johnson: *'A writer only begins a book. A reader finishes it.'* The authors of each of the subsequent chapters have shared examples of how the concept of One Health can be applied within veterinary nursing and how veterinary nurses have an essential and significant contribution to make. As already discussed, the concept of One Health is dynamic and continuously evolving, much like the veterinary nursing profession itself. It is therefore the editors' hope that readers will use the knowledge they gain from reading about the different aspects of One Health throughout this book and continually apply and evolve it as they progress through their careers.

Acknowledgements

The editors would like to express their gratitude to each of the authors who have contributed to this book. This book would not have been possible without their collective experience, knowledge and examples of their own practical application of One Health within their roles.

References

Capua, I. and Cattoli, G. (2018) One Health (r)Evolution: learning from the past to build a new future. *Viruses* 10(12), 725. doi: 10.3390/v10120725

Cook, R.A., Karesh, W.B. and Osofsky, S.A. (2004) The Manhattan Principles on 'One World, One Health'. *Conference summary. One World, One Health: Building interdisciplinary bridges to health in a globalized world*, 29 September, New York. Wildlife Conservation Society, New York, 29 September 2004 Symposium Available at: oneworldonehealth.org (accessed June, 2022)

Destoumieux-Garzon, D., Mavingui, P., Boetsch, G., Boissier, J., Darriet, F. *et al.* (2018) The One Health Concept: 10 years and a long road ahead. *Frontiers of Veterinary Science* 5, 14.

Evans, B.R. and Leighton, F.A. (2014) A history of One Health. *Revue Scientifique et Technique* 33(2), 413–420. doi: 10.20506/rst.33.2.2298

FAO/OIE/WHO (2010) *The FAO–OIE–WHO Collaboration. Sharing responsibilities and coordinating global activities to address health risks at the animal–*

human–ecosystems interfaces. A Tripartite Concept Note. Food and Agriculture Organization of the United Nations (FAO), World Organization for Animal Health (OIE) and World Health Organization (WHO). Available at: https://www.fao.org/3/ak736e/ak736e00.pdf (accessed June, 2022)

FAO/OIE/WHO (2017) *Providing multi-sectoral collaborative leadership in addressing health challenges.* Food and Agriculture Organization of the United Nations (FAO), World Organization for Animal Health (OIE) and World Health Organization (WHO). Available at: Tripartie2017f.pub (woah.org) (accessed June, 2022)

Gibbs, E.P.J. (2014) The evolution of One Health: a decade of progress and challenges for the future. *Veterinary Record* 174, 85–91. doi: org/10.1136/vr.g143

Joint Tripartite (FAO/OIE/WHO) and UNEP Statement (2021) *Tripartite and UNEP support OHHLEP's definition of One Health.* Available at: https://www.fao.org/3/cb7869en/cb7896en.pdf (accessed June, 2022)

Nelson, T., Kagan, N., Critchlow, C., Hillard, A. and Hsu, A. (2020) The danger of misinformation in the COVID-19 crisis. *Missouri Medicine* 117(6), 510–512.

One Health High Level Expert Panel (2021) *Annual Report.* Available at: https://cdn.who.int/media/docs/default-source/food-safety/onehealth/ohhlep-annual-report-2021.pdf (accessed June 2022)

The Human–Animal–Environment Interface

2

Rebecca Jones*
Langford Vets, Bristol, UK

Key Points

- The connections and interactions between humans, animals and the environment
- The impacts of anthropogenic activity
- Examples of issues faced at the human–animal–environment interface

2.1 Introduction

The fundamental concept of One Health is that humans, animals and the environment are intrinsically linked, sharing the planet through interdependent relationships (Evans and Leighton, 2014; Capua and Cattloli, 2018). The human–animal–environment (HAE) interface refers to the connections and interactions between this triad. This chapter provides an introduction to these relationships and some of the key issues faced at the human–animal–environment interface. It is a continuously evolving topic, but the key message is that the scope of veterinary nursing should not be restricted to just that of the animals under our care, or even to that of both the animals under our care and their owners. We also need to understand the world in which they live and the interactions they have with each other, other species and their environment and the impact that this can have on them all. The COVID-19 pandemic has been a stark reminder of just how important this is.

Since the 19th century and Industrial Period, human activity has been a dominant force and, while this has seen positive advancements in technology, industrialization and globalization among others, it has also had significant negative implications. This force has accelerated at a rate never

*Email: Becky.Jones@bristol.ac.uk

DOI: 10.1079/9781789249477.0002

previously seen in any other period in human history, leading to its unofficial recognition as the Anthropocene Epoch – the geological age of human impact on Earth (Myers *et al.*, 2013). The rate of environmental change is accelerating, negatively affecting environmental health and disrupting ecosystems and biodiversity that, in turn, impacts on the health and lives of all living species within it (see section 2.3, Anthropogenic Effects).

2.2　Infectious Diseases

The HAE interface is a source of emerging and re-emerging infectious diseases; approximately 75% of emerging infectious diseases are believed to be zoonotic (i.e. transmitted from animals to humans) with the majority of these originating from wild species (Jones *et al.*, 2008). This ability to jump species barriers is being made easier by factors such as the growing human population and the increasing proximity of humans and animals because of this. These diseases also have an increased ability to spread rapidly worldwide, due to increased global movement and trade (Jones *et al.*, 2008). COVID-19 is one such example and is the third beta-coronavirus to have crossed the animal–human species barrier within the past 20 years, resulting in a major zoonotic outbreak; the others being the causes of severe acute respiratory syndrome (SARS-CoV) and Middle East respiratory syndrome (MERS-CoV) (Schmiege *et al.*, 2020). Other notable infectious diseases considered to be public health emergencies of international concern include Ebola virus disease, Zika virus disease and influenza.

SARS was the first novel and severe infectious disease to emerge in the 21st century, subsequently followed by avian influenza H5N1, becoming a key driver for the 'One Health' approach of today and the increased recognition of the importance of a collaborative, cross-disciplinary approach in response to emerging and re-emerging infectious diseases (Mackenzie and Jeggo, 2019). Rabies is another high-profile zoonotic disease and is estimated to cause 59,000 deaths per year, mostly of children, despite being 100% preventable by vaccination, with 99% of human cases transmitted via dog bites (www.missionrabies.com, accessed March 2022). Campaigns to eliminate rabies in dogs via vaccination and to increase awareness and education of the disease, led by organizations such as Mission Rabies, are a great example of the impact of a One Health collaboration.

The changing HAE interface, notably increased global movement, has also affected the epidemiology of diseases in domestic animals that, although they may not have zoonotic potential, can still have a major socioeconomic impact. One such example is foot-and-mouth disease (FMD); the outbreak in the UK in 2001 had a devasting impact on agriculture and tourism (because of the media portrayal of the UK countryside being 'closed for business', an estimated 5.43 million UK consumers changed their travel plans due to the FMD outbreak (Leslie and Black, 2006)), resulting in the culling of over 6 million cows and sheep. The UK agriculture and industrial economic costs alone were estimated to be over £6 billion (Reperant *et al.*, 2012). Global movement has also contributed to an increase in non-endemic disease risks in companion animals, such as the recent increase in cases of *Brucella canis* in the UK, as a result of global movement of dogs to and from high-risk countries such as Romania (HAIRS, 2021). The continuing trend in popularity of exotic species as pets (Grant *et al.*, 2017) is another example further contributing to the variation and risk of infectious disease transmission.

Infectious diseases have a major impact on health systems, economies and society at a local, national and global level and therefore they continue to be a driving force for the One Health concept (see Chapter 5: Communicable Diseases). However, they are not the only threats faced; antimicrobial resistance, an increasing incumbrance of non-communicable diseases and food security and safety are other examples considered to be major global concerns (Evans and Leighton, 2014; Destoumieux-Garzon *et al.*, 2018).

In addition, these issues are interconnected and therefore it would be remiss to consider any of them in isolation. For example, antimicrobial resistance impacts both control of infectious diseases and food security and safety. Likewise, food insecurity impacts the lifestyles and nutrition of both humans and other animal species, notably companion animals, which has implications for the risks of developing non-communicable diseases. The effects of climate change, accelerated by human activity for the purpose of sustaining human life, now threaten the sustainability not just of human life but of all life on Earth.

2.3   Anthropogenic Effects

The term anthropogenic means caused by or influenced by human activity. In the past century, humans have altered the planet more rapidly and more extensively than any other comparable period in human history (Millennium Ecosystem Assessment, 2005; IPBES, 2019). This extensive alteration has seen many advancements, including the global indicators of health (Myers *et al.*, 2013). However, this progress has been reliant on many of the Earth's natural resources (see section 2.4: The Biosphere, Ecosystems and Biodiversity). As the human population continues to grow, so the demand on these resources also increases. Ultimately, this rate of progress cannot be sustained as these finite resources become depleted. In addition, the effect of this degradation is disproportionately affecting specific population groups, with poorer populations more vulnerable to the effects (Myers *et al.*, 2013). The human population now exceeds 7 billion and is expected to reach over 9 billion by 2050 (UN, 2019). This rapid growth has led to increased demands on food production and an increased requirement for land suitable for agricultural, industrial and residential purposes. Furthermore, it is anticipated that much of this global population increase will be concentrated in some of the least developed countries who are least resilient, further compounding the issues already faced (UN, 2019). Our planet can replenish over time but the rapid pace at which these resources are being exploited means that we are facing a global crisis.

Examples of anthropogenic activities include energy production, industrialization, food production, transportation and personal and domestic activities. Examples of the impacts of these activities include deforestation, pollution, diminishment of fossil fuels, global warming and climate change, disruption of ecosystems and loss of biodiversity.

Alterations to land represent some of the most extensive anthropogenic changes, including deforestation of approximately 50% of temperate and tropical forests and the conversion of 50% of terrestrial landscape to croplands or pasture (Myers *et al.*, 2013). This is closely followed by the over-exploitation of animals, plants and other organisms (mainly due to harvesting, logging, hunting and fishing), climate change, pollution and invasive species (IPBES, 2019). Direct exploitation of organisms, mostly due to fishing, and land/ sea use change have had the most significant impact on marine ecosystems (IPBES, 2019). These impacts, among others, are reducing biodiversity and distribution of natural ecosystems, disrupting their protective benefits, including water purification and retention, soil protection, pollination and climate regulation.

2.4   The Biosphere, Ecosystems and Biodiversity

The biosphere is made up of all parts of the Earth where living organisms exist. Within this biosphere exist many ecosystems – communities of living organisms (microorganisms, plants and animals) interacting with each other and their non-living environment. Individual ecosystems can vary greatly in size and can reside within larger ecosystems known as biomes. Examples of biomes include tropical forests, deserts, grassland and oceans, while examples of ecosystems within these may include rivers, sand dunes, ponds or coral reefs. Biodiversity refers to the variety and variability of all living life on Earth. This biodiversity is so abundant that new species are continually being discovered or are still to be discovered. However, as a result of anthropogenic activity, many species are also threatened with extinction. The IPBES (2019) report stated that 25% of all mammal, bird and amphibian species are at risk, with a 58% population decline of vertebrate species between 1970 and 2012.

Inherently, humans have interacted both directly and indirectly with various ecosystems since the beginning of human history. Ecosystems and their components – water, soil, nutrients and organisms – are integral to maintaining the health and wellbeing of humans and other species. These benefits are known as ecosystem services – the human utilization of resources produced by the environment.

Ecosystem services are classified as follows (adapted from the Millennium Ecosystem Assessment, 2005) (see also Fig. 2.1).

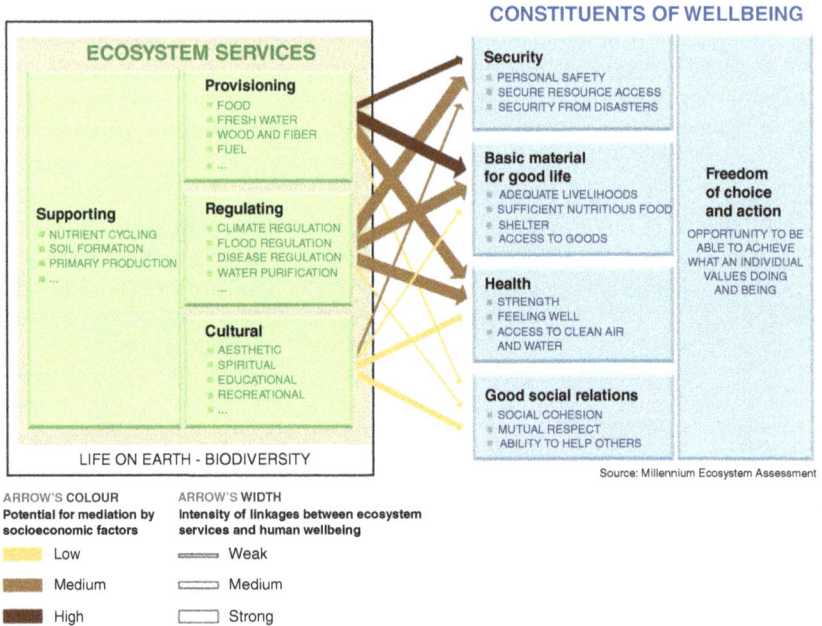

Fig. 2.1. The strength of linkages between commonly encountered categories of ecosystem services and components of human wellbeing (*Millennium Ecosystem Assessment*, 2005).

1. Provisioning Services. Products obtained from ecosystems include food, water, wood, biofuels, natural medicines and pharmaceuticals. Ecosystems provide the conditions for these resources to grow.

2. Regulating Services. Ecosystems act as regulators, for example of air quality, soil quality and greenhouse gases. Living organisms contribute to this regulation by assisting with pest and disease control.

3. Supporting Services. These form the foundation of ecosystems by providing the services required to sustain life, for example maintaining biodiversity, habitat provision and nutrient cycling.

4. Cultural Services. These are the non-material benefits such as recreation and opportunities for tourism, physical and mental health benefits, cultural identity and spiritual experience.

The Millennium Ecosystem Assessment (2005) was initiated in 2001 and was a 4-year process involving the collaborative work of 1360 experts worldwide. One of the objectives was to assess the consequences of ecosystem change for human wellbeing. One of their findings was that approximately 60% of ecosystems services examined were being degraded or used unsustainably. Most of the impacts of ecosystem change are due to an increased demand for food, water, timber and fuel. The Intergovernmental Science-Policy Platform on Biodiversity and Ecosystem Services Global Assessment on Biodiversity and Ecosystem Services (IPBES, 2019) reported a 75% alteration to land surface, 66% cumulative impacts to oceans, a loss of over 85% of wetlands and a 20% decline in the abundance of native species in most terrestrial biomes. It projected climate change to become a significant direct driver of increasing adverse changes to ecosystem services. The United Nations (UN) 2030 Agenda for Sustainable Development was adopted by all UN Member States in 2015 as a plan of action for people, planet and prosperity with the development of 17 Sustainable Development Goals (SDGs) and a call for action by all countries in a global partnership (UN, 2015). As part of this, it recognized that continued social and economic development and sustaining and improving human life depend on the sustainable management of these ecosystem services and the protection of the planet. All these reports can be accessed and are referenced at the end of this chapter.

2.5   Climate Change and Global Warming

Climate change is one of the most pressing global challenges faced. Climate change refers to the long-term shifts in average conditions such as ambient temperature and weather patterns, and the effects of these shifts, such as melting glaciers, increased rainfall and droughts, and rising sea levels. Global warming, also known as global heating, more starkly refers to the planet's rising surface temperature. The 'greenhouse effect' is the mechanism by which solar heat is trapped close to the Earth's surface by 'greenhouse gases', with this heat then being radiated back to Earth. It is so called as it has a protective 'greenhouse' effect, insulating the planet and preventing it from freezing. Greenhouse gases include carbon dioxide, methane, nitrous oxide and water vapour. These gases occur naturally but human activity has upset the balance, causing the concentration of gases in the atmosphere to increase, most significantly carbon dioxide, which in turn is causing the Earth's temperature to rise at exponential rates. Global surface temperature has increased faster since 1970 than in any other 50-year period over the past 2000 years (IPCC, 2021). Without a significant reduction in carbon dioxide and other greenhouse gases, global warming of 1.5°C and 2°C will be exceeded during the 21st century, with each incremental rise leading to more extreme weather events (IPCC, 2021). Impacts of climate change include changes in the distribution of infectious disease, in part through altered geographical distribution of vectors, food shortages due to seasonal changes, flooding, drought and natural disasters, and increased heat-related mortality in many species. Climate change is predicted to have a major impact on health, resulting in an estimated 250,000 additional global deaths per year between 2023 and 2050 (WHO, 2021).

Human activity has been accelerating climate change since the early 19th century when the Industrial period was well underway. This acceleration coincided with the switch to using fossil fuels to provide most of the world's energy, and while this contributed to great advancements in society, it also came at a cost. Of the 50 billion tonnes of greenhouse gases emitted into the world per year, energy production accounts for over 70% (Ritchie *et al.*, 2020).

In addition to the burning of fossil fuels, land use alterations, agriculture and forestry contribute to approximately 18.4% of global greenhouse gas emissions (Ritchie *et al.*, 2020). This includes an estimated contribution of up to 3% of global agricultural carbon emissions through pet food production (see Chapter 7, Environmental Sustainability in Veterinary Practice). Forests and soils act as carbon sinks, absorbing and storing carbon dioxide through photosynthesis. Land use alterations lead to deforestation and soil disruption. Forests remove a significant proportion of anthropogenic carbon dioxide emissions – a role that they cannot fulfil if destroyed. Soil disruption leads to erosion and leaching of nutrients, disrupting its ability to act as a carbon sink and causing the release of stored carbon dioxide back into the atmosphere. Nitrous oxide is produced when synthetic nitrogen fertilizers are applied to agricultural soils to increase productivity. Methane is produced by livestock, mainly cattle and sheep, through their digestive processes and both nitrous oxide and methane are produced from decomposing manure, especially in areas where large numbers of animals are confined such as on feed lots used for beef production (Ritchie *et al.*, 2020).

Climate change also has a significant impact on biodiversity, including affecting the timing of species life cycle events, altering species distributions and contributing to species extinction (Bellard *et al.*, 2012).

Even with action, the greenhouse gas emissions already released as a result of anthropogenic activity mean that some of the impacts of climate change will continue to be a concern for many decades to come (IPCC, 2021). As with all challenges faced under the One Health umbrella, how best to tackle climate change is complex and requires consideration of the social and political contexts as well as the science; we need to understand the issues from all perspectives (Victor, 2015). Chapter 7 (Environmental Sustainability in Veterinary Practice) provides further information and insight into how veterinary nurses can help to address climate change within their roles and practices.

2.6   Non-Communicable Diseases (NCDs)

According to the World Health Organization (WHO, 2021), NCDs are the cause of 71% of all global deaths. Both developed and developing countries face the double burden of infectious disease (also referred to as communicable disease) and non-communicable disease (i.e. diseases that cannot be transmitted from one organism to another, such as obesity, cardiovascular disease, cancer and diabetes mellitus), with an increasing prevalence of NCDs in developing countries (Boutayeb, 2010). As with infectious diseases, this increase is driven by anthropogenic changes but also factors often indicative of economic development, such as increased consumption of processed food, more sedentary lifestyles, changing cultural norms and the impacts of globalization and urbanization (Islam *et al.*, 2014). NCDs also represent a global socioeconomic burden and, as such, are recognized as a major challenge for the UN 2030 Agenda for Sustainable Development (WHO, 2021).

Environmental risk factors are shown to play an important role in NCDs in humans, with air pollution specifically being one of the greatest risks (Prüss-Ustün *et al.*, 2019; WHO, 2021). Other environmental risks include radiation, noise, climate change, pesticides, heavy metals and changing land use. An increasingly urban lifestyle is leading to an increased exposure to many of these risk factors. These risk factors are not restricted to humans and increase the risk of NCDs in many other species (Natterson-Horowitz *et al.*, 2022) (Fig. 2.2).

Epigenetics is the study of how external factors, such as nutrition and physical activity, and environmental factors can modify gene expression. Epigenetic changes can be maintained through cell division and have the potential to be transmitted to future generations (known as epigenetic transgenerational inheritance). Environmental factors, including nutrition and exposure to pollutants and toxicants (fungicides, pesticides and plastics), have been shown to promote epigenetic transgenerational inheritance of non-communicable diseases (Skinner, 2014). These transgenerational effects have been described in a variety of species, including wildlife (Destoumieux-Garzon *et al.*, 2018). For example, drought and temperature have been shown to be critical environmental factors for insects and plants (Skinner, 2014).

The comparative factors of non-communicable diseases in companion animals and their owners are explored further in Chapter 4 (Non-Communicable Diseases and Other Shared Health Risks).

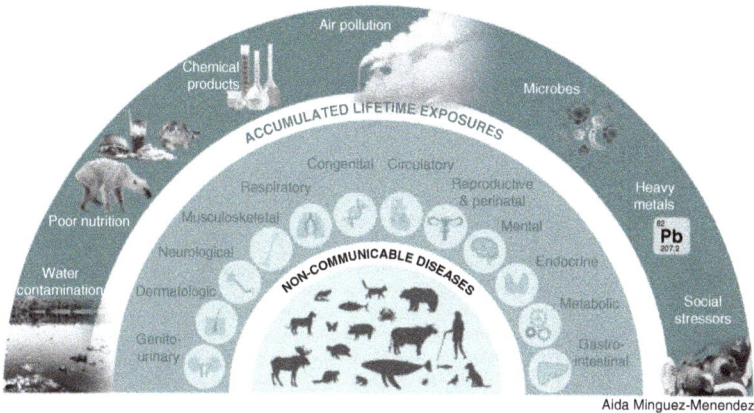

Aida Minguez-Menendez

Fig. 2.2. Shared environmental exposures contribute to NCDs across species. (Attributed to Natterson-Horowitz *et al.*, 2022, copyright Natterson-Horowitz, Desmarchelier, Winkler and Carabin; available for use under license CC BY.)

2.7   Antimicrobial Resistance (AMR)

Antimicrobial resistance is a major global concern for humans and animals. It is a naturally occurring phenomenon whereby, through random mutation or gene transfer, organisms acquire resistance to compounds secreted by other microorganisms that endows them with a survival advantage. Exposure to synthetic antimicrobials results in a similar selection pressure favouring AMR organisms and where these AMR organisms cause disease the antimicrobials are frequently ineffective. AMR organisms can be found in soil, water and air and can transfer between species, including within food supplies of animal origin, and are not limited by international borders. Although the existence of AMR precedes the discovery and use of antimicrobials, prevalence of AMR is increasing primarily through misuse and overuse of antimicrobials resulting in increased selection pressure. Environmental factors are also a concern, especially in areas where poor sanitation and limited access to clean water can increase vulnerability to contact with AMR organisms and antimicrobial compounds (WHO, 2021).

Many of the antimicrobials used to treat animals are the same as or similar to those for human use. The Food and Agriculture Organization of the UN reports that 27 different antimicrobial classes are used in animals (FAO, 2022). Globally, antimicrobials are heavily used in both agriculture and aquaculture. Quantifying total global use is challenging, due to poor surveillance and data collection in many countries. However, intensive farming methods have seen an increasing use of antimicrobials, with pig and cattle farms being the largest users (FAO, 2022). This is believed to be related to poor welfare conditions, increased stress and increased stocking densities of livestock, promoting the risk of disease. The use of antimicrobials in food-producing animals can also be transferred to humans and other animals via meat and animal products, presenting a food security and safety issue of concern. Environmental pollution as a result of excretions from both terrestrial and aquatic species and from manufacturing waste products further contributes to the global burden of AMR.

The accelerated emergence of AMR coincides with a decline in the discovery and development of new antimicrobials. It is therefore imperative that use of existing antimicrobials is safeguarded and there are many initiatives at global, national and local levels raising awareness of this issue and providing guidance on appropriate antimicrobial use. Veterinary nurses can play a key role in tackling the threat of AMR (see Chapter 5, Communicable Diseases).

Antimicrobials are not the only medicines of concern. The misuse and overuse of parasiticide products within livestock have been a concern for some time. More recently, concerns have been raised regarding their use within small animal medicine, relating to environmental contamination and their detrimental effect on wildlife and ecosystems (Perkins *et al.*, 2021; BVA, 2022). Further research is still ongoing in this area.

2.8   Food Production, Food Security and Food Safety

One of the drivers behind anthropogenic change is the increasing requirement for food. Agriculture and the domestication of animals for food and other purposes are believed to have begun around 12,000 years ago, during the period of the neolithic revolution. This transition from the hunter-gatherer period to permanent settlements, with the ability to farm crops and animals, saw civilizations established and human populations rapidly increase. As mentioned, the human population is expected to reach over 9 billion by 2050. To support this, food production is predicted to need to increase by 50% from 2012 production levels, placing additional strain on the challenge to provide safe and nutritious food for the population (Garcia *et al.*, 2020). Already, approximately 11% of the world's population is believed to be undernourished, with a 20% associated mortality rate (IPBES, 2019).

2.8.1   Food production

The increasing demands for food have led to radical changes to the way in which it is produced and supplied. Many elements of our current food systems are unsustainable, contributing to loss of biodiversity, deforestation, water scarcity and soil degradation, having a significant impact on the health of the planet. Agricultural expansion accounts for over one-third of terrestrial land surface being used for crops and animal husbandry (IPBES, 2019). Changes in land use for food production and the encroachment into wildlife habitats are increasing domestic animal and wildlife interactions, providing new opportunities for emerging and re-emerging disease transmission. Alongside this, more intensive farming methods and high stocking densities of livestock are contributing to welfare issues and increased risk of disease. It is not just terrestrial food production that is having an impact: fish are a major source of the world's protein. Anthropogenic changes have had a widespread impact on oceans, most notably over-exploitation of fish, shellfish and other organisms, but also because of land/sea-based pollution and land/sea use alterations, such as coastal development (IPBES, 2019). Food production, whether from land or from water, is dependent on a healthy planet and functioning ecosystems; without these, food production cannot be sustained, let alone increase.

The responsibility on food producers to meet supply demands, providing nutrient- and energy-rich food, while also ensuring food security and safety, presents a challenging and complex problem with objectives at conflict with each other, but an increasing number of initiatives are being developed. Definitions of 'sustainable' agriculture techniques vary and are often synonymous; however, examples of techniques being employed include soil and water conservation practices (such as reduced soil tilling), reducing use of pesticides and synthetic fertilizers, and integrated crop and livestock production systems. Soil health and water preservation are significant; healthy soil is fundamental for healthy, nutritious food, and crops and livestock reportedly already account for 70% of all global water withdrawals (FAO, 2017). Regenerative agriculture is gaining popularity and has been proposed as a step on from sustainable agriculture – a term used to describe a combination of techniques aimed at not just sustaining but restoring agricultural ecosystems. It employs five key principles: (i) reducing soil disturbance; (ii) protecting the soil by improving soil coverage; (iii) ensuring living roots in the soil all year round; (iv) practising crop diversity; and (v) integrating livestock. A range of claims have been made regarding the ability of regenerative agriculture to enhance the health of soil and increase its productivity and the positive impact that this could have on climate change and biodiversity, but these claims have still to be substantiated.

2.8.2   Food security

Food security has been defined by the FAO (FAO *et al.*, 2021) as a situation that exists '*when all people, at all times, have physical, social and economic access to sufficient, safe and nutritious food that meets their dietary needs and food preferences for an active and healthy life*'.

The number of people affected by food insecurity has been slowly increasing since 2015, meaning that zero hunger (the UN's Sustainable Development Goal (SDG) 2) is not on track to be achieved (FAO *et al.*, 2021). The higher costs of healthy diets versus income inequality amongst populations means that millions of people worldwide cannot afford to eat nutritious food, leaving them vulnerable to different forms of malnutrition, such as nutrient deficiencies and obesity, contributing further to the escalating global burden of non-communicable diseases (FAO *et al.*, 2021). There is no single nationwide government measure for food insecurity in the UK, but it is believed that the number of people in the UK experiencing hunger is growing. Recently published data (Food Foundation, 2022) indicates a continuing rise in food insecurity in the UK, affecting approximately 8.8% of households (4.7 million adults and 2 million children). People with disabilities and those in receipt of social security payments (Universal Credit) are reported to be five times more at risk.

The extent to which companion animals are affected by food insecurity is much harder to quantify. To date, companion animals are not included in national household surveys relating to this topic. Given their shared lifestyles and living environments, it should be considered that the animals in a household affected by food insecurity will be affected too. A study by Arluke (2021) showed that pet food insecurity existed, with respondents indicating that this was a cause of emotional distress and needing to resort to coping mechanisms such as feeding less, sharing their own food or relying on food banks and goodwill of neighbours and family to feed their pet. Rauktis *et al.* (2017) reported similar findings with regard to owners sharing their own food with their pets. Interestingly, a further study by Rauktis *et al.* (2020) indicated a positive link between pet ownership and maintaining the owner's food security, with the suggestion that pets can create a motivation to obtain food. They suggested the benefits of food banks that cater for both humans and animals. These studies highlight the interlinks of the human–animal bond: owners will often put their animals' needs before their own and this can have consequences for both their own nutritional status and that of their pets. It again raises the benefits of a One Health approach – collaborative and multidisciplinary thinking – when tackling issues such as food insecurity.

Climate change, accelerated by anthropogenic activity, is amplifying natural disasters. Natural disasters, such as hurricanes, floods, earthquakes and wildfires, pose a significant threat to food security by impacting on food production and availability in several ways: loss of animals and crops, destruction of agricultural infrastructure, and environmental contamination with pathogens, chemicals and other pollutants (Garcia *et al.*, 2020). Infectious disease and human-induced disasters, such as conflict, political instability and other socioeconomic crises, are additional drivers of food insecurity with more than half of people who are undernourished living in countries experiencing conflict or fragility (FAO *et al.*, 2021). According to FAO *et al.* (2021), approximately 30 million more people may face hunger in 2030 than if the COVID-19 pandemic had not occurred, an example of the impact and long-lasting effects of such an event.

Increasing food production is not the only solution in tackling food security. FAO (2013) estimated that approximately one-third of the world's food produced is lost or wasted every year. This is not only a significant economic waste: food waste also contributes to greenhouse gas emissions and climate change.

2.8.3   Food safety

Globalization has resulted in an increased demand for a wider variety of food sources, which has led to an increasingly complex global food chain and further amplified the risk of foodborne disease outbreaks (WHO, 2022), with food sources able to become contaminated at many points in the process, including production and distribution. According to WHO (2022), an estimated 600 million people become ill after eating contaminated food, with 420,000 dying every year.

Foodborne disease can enter the body via contaminated food and water. Examples include: bacteria such as *Salmonella* spp., *Campylobacter* spp., *Escherichia coli* and *Listeria* spp.; viruses such as noroviruses and Hepatitis A; and parasites such as the *Echinoccoccus* spp. tapeworms, *Cryptosproidium* spp. and *Giardia* spp. Toxins and pollutants are also a growing concern, some of which are naturally occurring but others, such as persistent organic pollutants (POPs) are by-products of industrial processes and waste. Heavy metals such as lead and mercury can also contaminate food sources through pollution of air, water and soil. Pet food can also present a food safety concern. Commercial pet food diets, including treats, can serve as a vehicle for infectious disease, as well as toxicants, for both pets and their owners (Buchanan *et al.*, 2011). The increasing trend for raw food diets further contributes to this risk (Groat *et al.*, 2022) (see Chapter 5: Communicable Diseases).

Successful implementation of measures that can reduce the incidence and burden of foodborne disease is dependent on not only knowledge of the drivers and occurrence of these diseases but also an understanding and consideration of the socioeconomic context of key stakeholders, such as farmers, traders and consumers (Boqvist *et al.*, 2018).

2.9 Wildlife

Anthropogenic activity is having a significant impact on wildlife and although there are some positive effects of this, the impact is largely negative. The large-scale activities that are having the biggest impact, some of which have already been discussed, include alterations in land use and deforestation, resulting in loss of habitat and species decline, pollution, exploitation of many species (for example for fur, medicine, food and as pets) and introduction of new (sometimes invasive) species. There are other examples such as recreational activities, including hiking, climbing, boating, fishing and picnicking, that may be considered less of an issue but can have a significant cumulative ecological impact if not appropriately managed; the magnitude of the effects is influenced by many factors, including type, frequency, timing and location (Steidl and Powell, 2006).

The following are some examples of the impact of human activity on wildlife.

2.9.1 Human–wildlife interactions

Human–wildlife interactions vary from positive to negative, minor to severe, with frequency also variable within and among geographical regions (Nyhus, 2016). The term 'human–wildlife conflict' encompasses the negative interactions that occur between both people and their associated activities and the non-domesticated animals within their environment (Nyhus, 2016). This conflict occurs when the needs and behaviours of wildlife impact negatively on humans, or vice versa, and is reported to be one of the most complex issues facing wildlife and conservation management (Mekonen, 2020). Throughout their history, humans have competed with wildlife for food and resources, domesticated many species of animal while simultaneously eradicating others (both deliberately and accidentally), and employed a range of social, behavioural and technical approaches to manage their interactions with wildlife (Nyhus, 2016). We have already discussed the numerous negative impacts that human activity is having on wildlife, but human–wildlife conflict can have significant consequences for humans too. For example, wildlife species have the potential to destroy crops, resulting directly or indirectly (via spread of infectious disease) in famine, or killing and injuring of livestock resulting in loss of livelihood, and killing or injuring humans. This often means that the presence of some wildlife species may not be well tolerated, putting them under threat.

Conflict between humans and wildlife has been strongly linked to the decline of many animal species, resulting in ecological consequences for other species and ecosystem services (Nyhus, 2016). In particular, apex predators (i.e., those at the top of the food chain) are reported to be instrumental in shaping ecosystems (Ritchie *et al.*, 2012). There is a growing global interest in the reintroduction of apex predators (for example, the reintroduction of the lynx or wolf into Great Britain) and restoring native predator populations has also been reported as a potential natural solution to controlling invasive species (Ritchie *et al.*, 2012; Twining *et al.*, 2022). However, reintroduction schemes are not without controversy, with concerns regarding the impact of this reintroduction on the safety of other species, notably livestock and humans. There are also knowledge gaps relating to the effects that predators can have on the structure and function of ecosystems, as these effects do not work in isolation but are part of a more complex process, including the productivity of ecosystems and the diversity of species within them (Ritchie *et al.*, 2012).

There is the suggestion that using the phrase 'human–wildlife conflict' is not helpful in managing the co-existence of humans, domestic animals and wildlife and the term could, in fact, perpetuate the anthropomorphism of wildlife with the belief that these species are consciously antagonistic (Peterson *et al.*, 2010). It is important to recognize that the increasing contact between these species is because of the growing impingement of humans on the lives of wildlife, forcing wildlife species to adapt to survive. The use of the word 'conflict' also frames these interactions negatively, even when positive benefits can exist; therefore, there is growing convergence regarding the phrase 'human–wildlife conflict' and the suggestion that 'human–wildlife co-existence' or similar would be more appropriate, in recognition of both the issues and the solutions (Nyhus, 2016; Mekonen, 2020).

Regardless of the term used, the interactions between humans and wildlife present significant and complex issues for all and therefore form an important part of the conservation agenda with the recognition that appropriate solutions are dependent on understanding the complexities faced and involving and obtaining cooperation between all stakeholders. Human–wildlife interactions have potential impacts for many of UN SDGs (Gross *et al.*, 2021). A joint report by the World Wide Fund for Nature (WWF) and the UN Environment Programme (UNEP) – A Future for All: The Need for Human-Wildlife Coexistence (Gross *et al.*, 2021) – aims to raise the profile of the issues faced and the potential solutions.

2.9.2 The wildlife trade

The international wildlife trade poses a major threat to wild species worldwide, including threatened and endangered species. Both legal and illegal trades exist, with sometimes a blurring of the two. Because of this, and because wildlife may be traded as parts rather than whole, it is difficult to quantify the numbers of animals traded. However, it is believed that a quarter of the world's species are traded, legally or illegally. Birds are the most traded group of species, with an estimated 85% of these being traded as pets (Ritchie and Roser, 2021). Pangolins, also known as scaly anteaters, are reportedly the world's most trafficked. Wildlife and live animal markets occur in many parts of the world, including Southeast Asia, India, North and Latin America, Africa and Europe, and involve the trade of live animals and the derivatives from wild-caught or captive-bred non-domesticated animals for fashion, traditional medicine, culinary and pet trades (Warwick and Steedman, 2021). The impacts of this trade are multifactorial and include significant threats to species conservation, removal of large numbers of animals from indigenous habitats, inhumane practices, and severe deprivation of animal husbandry and welfare needs. The stress induced by these conditions, and consequential sustained increase in cortisol, increases susceptibility to disease. This, along with high stocking densities, accumulation of waste products and diverse mixing of species, added to the high density of human populations often present at these markets, presents many opportunities for infectious disease spillover (Warwick and Steedman, 2021).

It is important to differentiate between the different types of markets that are commonplace across many parts of the world. The term 'wet market', for example, is often misunderstood. These markets came under intense scrutiny at the start of the COVID-19 pandemic, with a hypothesis that the virus originated from a 'wet market' in Wuhan, China. While it is true that some wet markets do sell live animals, including wildlife species (as was the case in Wuhan), many wet markets sell only fresh seafood, meat and vegetables. They get their name from the ice, used to keep food fresh, melting and causing the floors to become slick with water. Local communities depend upon such markets for food, income and social cohesion and there is a need to understand the cultural and socioeconomic aspects of these markets and their role in food security alongside solutions to address the issues of animal welfare, poor sanitation and disease risks (Naguib et al., 2021).

There has been such a large decline in wildlife populations, due to hunting and poaching, that some areas of the world are referred to as 'empty ecosystems'; the bushmeat trade alone is estimated to have caused a 60% decline in species populations, with a selective loss of large mammals and primates, changing the dynamics of ecosystems (Ritchie and Roser, 2021). Bushmeat is the term used to describe the meat from wild animals killed in the forests and savannahs, primarily of Africa. Bushmeat is a valuable source of protein, with many rural communities relying on the hunting of wildlife for food as the farming of domesticated animals is too expensive or impractical. There is cor-relation between food insecurity and wildlife consumption; in the absence of other food sources, communities come to rely on wildlife for food, particularly as a source of protein and fat. There is also correlation between the consump-tion of bushmeat and the transmission of infectious diseases; the hunting, gathering and butchering of wild meat presents a high risk of blood-borne dis-ease transmission such as Ebola virus disease and human immunodeficiency virus (HIV) (Ritchie and Roser, 2021). The bushmeat trade is an example of a growing wildlife trade and is very different to the hunting of wildlife by rural communities for food security. The increase in this trade is linked to multiple factors, including population growth, increased access to areas because of deforestation and land development, improvements in hunting technology, and its popularity as a status symbol for urban populations. This trade is con-sidered a significant threat to wildlife, affecting many species, including goril-las and other primates, elephants, antelope, crocodiles and fruit bats. This loss of wildlife contributes to biodiversity decline and further degradation of the ecosystem.

The wildlife trade does not just involve animal species; many plant spe-cies are both legally and illegally traded. Since 1975, 1.8 billion exports of plants have been reported (Ritchie and Roser, 2021). The illegal trade in tim-ber is another example and one which is further contributing to the defores-tation and destruction of habitats. The Convention on International Trade in Endangered Species of Wild Fauna and Flora (CITES) is the principal global framework regulating the international wildlife trade. This is an international voluntary agreement between governments, including the UK, with the aim of ensuring that international trade does not threaten the survival of species; it provides varying degrees of protection to more than 37,000 species of animals and plants. It does, however, have significant limitations regarding enforce-ment as well as several loopholes such as traceability of the origins of species. As such, the illegal wildlife trade continues to grow, reportedly being the fourth biggest illegal trade in the world and worth over an estimated £17 billion a year. This illegal trade is also closely linked with organized crime syndicates involved in other criminal activity such as arms, drugs and human traffick-ing. The UK is both a transit and destination country for the wildlife trade and therefore instrumental in tackling the global illegal wildlife trade. The role of the UK National Wildlife Crime Unit (NWCU) (available at www.nwcu.police. uk, accessed March 2022) is to assist in the prevention and detection of wildlife crime, including the trade in species protected under CITES. Their other key UK priorities are:

- Persecution of badgers and bats
- Poaching
- Persecution of raptors – poisoning, egg and chick theft, removing from the wild, and nest disturbance/destruction
- Cyber-enabled wildlife crime – much of the UK wildlife trade is conducted via online platforms opening the trade to a global market.

One example of an NWCU national campaign is Operation Easter, which targets thieves of rare wild bird eggs as well as tackling the online trade in eggs and the disturbance and destruction of nests.

2.9.3 Non-native and invasive species

Non-native or introduced species (including animals, plants and fungi) are those found outside their normal range because of human activity, while those that have a negative effect on native species or the environment into which they are introduced are also described as invasive. Not all introduced species are detrimental. Non-native species can be moved by humans deliberately (for example livestock, such as pigs, sheep and goats for food; cats and dogs for predation and protection) or inadvertently (for example rats gaining carriage to non-native regions on boats; plant or seeds carried on clothes or in cargo). Invasive species have increased by 40% since 1980 because of increased global movement, trade and expanding human populations with nearly one-fifth of the Earth's surface at risk (IPBES, 2019). Within the UK, there are estimated to be more than 3000 non-native species, including the grey squirrel, mink, muntjac deer, Asian hornet and Japanese knotweed. Invasive species are reported to pose one of the greatest global threats to biodiversity (Twining *et al.*, 2022). The consequences for native species are multifactorial and include predation, competition, introduction of new diseases and impacts on genetic diversity because of hybrid breeding. Invasive species also contribute to the complexities of human–wildlife conflict, as detailed above.

2.10   Urbanization

The most recent projections from the UN (UN-Habitat, 2020) suggest that urban areas will house 68% of the global population by 2050. Currently, urban areas cover less than 3% of total land area, but this is expected to triple by 2030 (IPBES, 2019). Developing countries are expected to experience the most significant growth, with a projected 90% of the population growth expected to occur within urban areas (Hassell *et al.*, 2017).

There are 'push' and 'pull' factors behind the increase in urbanized populations. Push factors are those that promote movement *away* from an area and pull factors are those that promote movement *into* an area. Examples of factors include job opportunities, living conditions, access to education and health services and avoidance of natural disasters or war and conflict. However, urbanization is another example of how rapid development cannot sustain the benefits equally for all. The UN-Habitat's *World Cities Report* (2020) states that well-planned and well-managed urbanization can vastly improve quality of life for all, but unplanned urbanization leaves people vulnerable. The COVID-19 pandemic exposed and exacerbated the significant inequalities between different

groups, notably those inequalities negatively affecting the poorer populations, due to uneven access to healthcare, inadequate housing and sanitation
and precarious employment security (UN-Habitat, 2020). The risks of non-
communicable diseases are increased in urban areas, due to unhealthy living
and working conditions secondary to inadequate access to green space, urban
heat island effects and exposure to pollution being more prevalent in urban
areas (WHO, 2021). Although less is known about the effects of urbanization on the health of companion animals, there is evidence to suggest similar
links as for humans (Hakanen *et al.*, 2018; Natterson-Horowitz *et al.*, 2022).
Urbanization is a driver for increasing contacts between wildlife, humans and
domesticated animals which increases the risk of disease spillover (Hassell
et al., 2017). Infectious diseases can also thrive and spread more rapidly in
urban areas, especially in areas with overcrowding and poor waste management (WHO, 2021).

Urbanization further contributes to environmental degradation, with significant impact on ecosystems and biodiversity due to habitat fragmentation
and loss. Evidence suggests that urbanization can have a significant impact
on wildlife communities, with biodiversity overall decreasing but with an
increasing proportion of species that are able to adapt to changes in altered
habitats and resource availability (Hassell *et al.*, 2017). There is also a significant pull on nature's resources with large generation of waste as a result,
further contributing to air, water and soil degradation. The urban heat island
effect refers to the higher temperatures experienced within urban areas, compared with rural areas, because of infrastructure development displacing
natural surfaces such as trees and soils, which act as moderators for temperature. As a result of these higher temperatures, infrastructures and vehicles
also consume more energy, which further exacerbates air pollution and climate change.

Green spaces (areas such as grass, trees and vegetation) and blue spaces
(visible water such as sea, rivers, lakes and canals) are a vital consideration
of urban planning, combating negative effects of urbanization such as air
pollution and the urban heat island effect, as well as having mental and
physical health benefits for those who use them (Anguluri and Narayanan,
2017). Public Health England (2020) reported that the removal of air pollution by urban green and blue spaces in the UK in 2017 equated to a saving
of £162.6 million in health costs. However, rapid urban expansion can make
it increasingly challenging to provide sufficient green and blue spaces. This
is another issue that highlights disparities between high- and low-income
populations. For example, the proportion of England's urban areas made up
of green spaces has declined and it is estimated that just 35% of households
in the lowest earning income bracket are within a 10-minute walk of pub-
licly accessible green space (Environment Agency UK, 2021). In England and
Wales, houses and flats within 100 metres of public green space are an average £2500 more expensive than they would be if 500 metres away (Public
Health England, 2020).

2.11   Summary

The issues faced at the human–animal interface are numerous and complex. Human activity has led to many advancements within civilization but at a great cost to our planet and the living species within it. The term 'human activity' can imply that all humans are equally responsible but many of the issues faced highlight and contribute to the growing inequities and disparities between populations and countries. It can be easy to condemn and judge situations that we do not fully understand. A One Health approach that can truly have a positive impact is dependent on understanding the issues faced through all lenses and understanding that actions can also have consequences. Education is key but we need to recognize that this education is a two-way process: to educate others, we first must educate ourselves. The global society in which we now live means that we need to recognize how the actions that we take and the decisions that we make in our roles can have an impact on the wider issues faced under the One Health umbrella. We are all connected.

2.12   Questions for Further Discussion

1. Consider the local community in which you work. How are the issues discussed in this chapter relevant and how can your role as a veterinary nurse have an impact?
2. What potential is there for transdisciplinary collaboration on the issues faced under One Health between veterinary nurses and other organizations within your local community?
3. As this chapter was being written, the war that commenced in February 2022 between Russia and Ukraine was still ongoing. Consider the impact that this war is having on the issues faced under One Health.

References

Anguluri, R. and Narayanan, P. (2017) Role of green space in urban planning: outlook towards smart cities. *Urban Forestry and Urban Greening* 25, 58–65.

Arluke, A. (2021) Coping with pet food insecurity in low-income communities. *Anthrozoos* 34(3), 339–358.

Bellard, C., Bertelsmeier, C., Leadley, P., Thuiller, W. and Courchamp, F. (2012) Impacts of climate change on the future of biodiversity. *Ecology Letters* 15(4), 365–377. doi: 10.1111/j.1461-0248.2011.01736.x

Boqvist, S., Söderqvist, K. and Vågsholm, I. (20180 Food safety challenges and One Health within Europe. *Acta Veterinaria Scandinavica* 60(1), 1.

Boutayeb, A. (2010) The burden of communicable and non-communicable diseases in developing countries. In: Preedy, V.R. and Watson, R.R. (eds) *Handbook of Disease Burdens and Quality of Life Measures*. Springer, New York, pp. 531–546.

Buchanan, R., Baker, R., Charlton, A., Riviere, J. and Standaert, R. (2011) Pet food safety: a shared concern. *British Journal of Nutrition* 106(S1), S78–S84.

BVA (2022) *Our policies. Responsible use of parasiticides for cats and dogs.* British Veterinary Association. Available at: www.bva.co.uk/take-action/our-policies/responsible-use-of-parasiticides-for-cats-and-dogs (accessed June 2022).

Capua, I. and Cattoli, G. (2018) One Health (r)Evolution: Learning from the past to build a new future. *Viruses* 10(12), 725. doi: 10.3390/v10120725

Destoumieux-Garzon, D., Mavingui, P., Boetsch, G., Boissier, J., Darriet, F. *et al.* (2018) The One Health Concept: 10 years and a long road ahead. *Frontiers of Veterinary Science* 5, 14.

Environment Agency UK, Chief Scientist's Group (2021) *The State of the Environment: The Urban Environment.* Environment Agency, Bristol, UK.

Evans, B.R. and Leighton, F.A. (2014) A history of One Health. *Revue Scientifique et Technique* 33(2), 413–420. doi: 10.20506/rst.33.2.2298.

FAO (2013) *Food wastage footprint: impacts on natural resources – summary report.* Food and Agriculture Organization of the United Nations, Rome. Available at: www.fao.org/3/i3347e/i3347e.pdf (accessed December 2022).

FAO (2017) *Water Pollution from Agriculture: A Global Review. Executive Summary.* Food and Agriculture Organization of the United Nations, Rome. Available at: https://www.fao.org/3/i7754e/i7754e.pdf (accessed December 2022).

FAO (2022) *Antimicrobial resistance.* Food and Agriculture Organization of the United Nations, Rome. Available at: https://www.fao.org/antimicrobial-resistance (accessed June 2022).

FAO, IFAD, UNICEF, WFP and WHO (2021) *The State of Food Security and Nutrition in the World 2021. Transforming food systems for food security, improved nutrition and affordable healthy diets for all.* Food and Agriculture Organization of the United Nations, Rome.

Food Foundation (2022) *Food Insecurity Tracking.* Available at: https://foodfoundation.org.uk/initiatives/food-insecurity-tracking (accessed February 2022).

Garcia, S.N., Osburn, B.I. and Jay-Russell, M.T. (2020) One Health for food safety, food security and sustainable food production. *Frontiers in Sustainable Food Systems* 4, 1. doi: 10.3389/fsufs.2020.00001

Grant, R.A., Montrose, V.T. and Wills, A.P. (2017) ExNOTic: should we be keeping exotic pets? *Animals* 7(6), 47. doi: 10.3390/ani7060047

Groat, E.F., Williams, N.J., Pinchbeck, G., Warner, B., Simpson, A. and Schmidt, V.M. (2022) UK dogs eating raw meat diets have higher risk of *Salmonella* and antimicrobial-resistant *Escherichia coli* faecal carriage. *Journal of Small Animal Practice* 63, 435–441. doi: 10.1111/jsap.13488

Gross, E., Jayasinghe, N., Brooks, A., Polet, G., Wadhwa, R. and Hilderink-Koopmans, F. (2021) *A Future for All: The Need for Human–Wildlife Coexistence.* World Wildlife Fund, Gland, Switzerland.

HAIRS (2021) *Risk Statement: Brucella canis.* Human Animal Infections and Risk Surveillance group. Available at: www.gov.uk/government/publications/hairs-risk-statement-brucella-canis (accessed June 2022).

Hakanen, E., Lehtimäki, J., Salmela, E., Tiira, K., Anturaniemi, J. *et al.* (2018) Urban environment predisposes dogs and their owners to allergic symptoms. *Scientific Reports* 8, 1585. doi: 10.1038/s41598-018-19953-3

Hassell, J.M., Begon, M., Ward, M.J. and Fèvre, E.M. (2017) Urbanization and disease emergence: dynamics at the wildlife–livestock–human interface. *Trends in Ecology & Evolution* 32(1), 55–67. doi: 10.1016/j.tree.2016.09.012

IPBES (2019) *Global assessment report on biodiversity and ecosystem services of the Intergovernmental Science-Policy Platform on Biodiversity and Ecosystem Services* (eds Brondizio, E.S., Settele, J., Díaz, S. and Ngo, H.T.). IPBES Secretariat, Bonn, Germany. doi: 10.5281/zenodo.3831673

IPCC (2021) Summary for Policymakers. In: Masson-Delmotte, V., Zhai, P., Pirani, A., Connors, S.L., Péan, S. *et al.* (eds) *Climate Change 2021: The Physical Science Basis.* Contribution of Working Group I to the Sixth Assessment Report of the Intergovernmental Panel on Climate Change. [In press.]

Islam, S.M., Purnat, T.D., Phuong, N.T., Mwingira, U., Schacht, K. and Fröschl, G. (2014) Non-communicable diseases (NCDs) in developing countries: a symposium report. *Global Health* 11(10), 81. doi: 10.1186/s12992-014-0081-9

Jones, K.E., Patel, N.G., Levy, M.A., Storeygard, A., Balk, D. *et al.* (2008) Global trends in emerging infectious diseases. *Nature* 451(7181), 990–993.

Leslie, D. and Black, L. (2006) Tourism and the impact of the foot and mouth epidemic in the UK. *Journal of Travel and Tourism Marketing* 19, 2–3, 35–46. doi: 10.1300/J073v19n02_04

Mackenzie, J.S. and Jeggo, M. (2019) The One Health approach – why is it so important? *Tropical Medicine and Infectious Disease* 4(2), 88.

Mekonen, S. (2020) Coexistence between human and wildlife: the nature, causes and mitigations of human wildlife conflict around Bale Mountains National Park, Southeast Ethiopia. *BMC Ecology* 20, 51. doi: org/10.1186/s12898-020-00319-1

Millennium Ecosystem Assessment (2005) *Ecosystems and Human Well-being: Synthesis.* World Resources Institute, Washington, DC.

Myers, S., Gaffkin, L., Golden, C.D., Ostfeld, R.S., Redford, K.H. *et al.* (2013) Human health impacts of ecosystem alteration. *Proceedings of the National Academy of Sciences of the USA* 110(47), 18753–18760. doi: 10.1073/pnas.1218656110

Naguib, M., Li, R., Ling, J., Grace, D., Nguyen-Viet, H. and Lindahl, J. (2021) Live and wet markets: food access versus the risk of disease emergence. *Trends in Microbiology* 29(7), 573–581. doi: 10.1016/j.tim.2021.02.007

Natterson-Horowitz, B., Desmarchelier, M., Winkler, A.S. and Carabin, H. (2022) Beyond zoonoses in One Health: Non-communicable diseases across the animal kingdom. *Frontiers in Public Health* 9, 807186.

Nyhus, P.J. (2016) Human–wildlife conflict and coexistence. *Annual Review of Environment and Resources* 41(1), 143–171.

Perkins, R., Whitehead, M., Civil, W. and Goulson, D. (2021) Potential role of veterinary flea products in widespread pesticide contamination of English rivers. *Science of the Total Environment* 755(1), 143560. doi: 10.1016/j.scitotenv.2020.143560

Peterson, M.N., Birckhead, J.L., Leong, K., Peterson, M.J. and Peterson, T.R. (2010) Rearticulating the myth of human–wildlife conflict. *Conservation Letters* 3, 74–82.

Prüss-Ustün, A., van Deventer, E., Mudu, P., Campbell-Lendrum, D., Vickers, C. *et al.* (2019) Environmental risk and non-communicable disease. *BMJ* 364, 1265.

Public Health England (2020) *Improving access to greenspace. A new review for 2020.* Available at: https://assets.publishing.service.gov.uk/government/uploads/system/uploads/attachment_data/file/904439/Improving_access_to_greenspace_2020_review.pdf (accessed January 2023).

Rauktis, M.E., Rose, L., Chen, Q., Martone, R. and Martello, A. (2017) 'Their pets are loved members of their family': Animal ownership, food insecurity, and the value of having pet food available in food banks. *Anthrozoös* 30(4), 581–593.

Rauktis, M.E., Lee, H., Bickel, L., Giovengo, H., Nagel, M. and Cahalane, H. (2020) Food Security Challenges and Health Opportunities of Companion Animal Ownership for Low-Income Adults. *Journal of Evidence-Based Social Work* 17(6), 662–676. doi: 10.1080/26408066.2020.1781726

Reperant, L.A., Cornaglia, G. and Osterhaus, A.D.M.E. (2012) The importance of understanding the human–animal interface. In: Mackenzie, J., Jegg, M., Daszak, P. and Richt, J. (eds) One Health: the human–animal–environment interfaces in emerging and infectious diseases. *Current Topics in Microbiology and Immunology*, Vol. 365. Springer, Berlin, Heidleberg.

Ritchie, E.G., Elmhagen, B., Glen, A.S., Letnic, M., Ludwig, G. and McDonald, R.A. (2012) Ecosystem restoration with teeth: what role for predators? *Trends in Ecology & Evolution* 27(5), 265–271. doi: 10.1016/j.tree.2012.01.001

Ritchie, H. and Roser, M. (2021) *Biodiversity*. Available at: https://ourworldindata.org/biodiversity (accessed June 2022)

Ritchie, H., Roser, M. and Rosado, P. (2020) *CO$_2$ and Greenhouse Gas Emissions*. Available at: https://ourworldindata.org/co2-and-other-greenhouse-gas-emissions (accessed June 2022).

Schmiege, D., Arredondo, A., Ntajal, J., Minetto, J., Paris, G. *et al.* (2020) One Health in the context of coronavirus outbreaks: a systematic literature review. *One Health* 10, 2352–7714. doi: 10.1016/j.onehlt.2020.100170

Skinner, M.K. (2014) Environmental stress and epigenetic transgenerational inheritance. *BMC Medicine* 12, 153

Steidl, R.J. and Powell, B.F. (2006) Assessing the effects of human activities on wildlife. *The George Wright Forum* 23(2), 50–58.

Twining, J.P., Lawton, C., White, A., Sheehy, E., Hobson, K. *et al.* (2022) Restoring vertebrate predator populations can provide landscape-scale biological control of established invasive vertebrates: Insights from pine marten recovery in Europe. *Global Change Biology* 00, 1–17.i. doi: 10.1111/gcb.16236

UN (2015) *Transforming Our World: the 2030 Agenda for Sustainable Development. United Nations Department of Economic and Social Affairs: Division for Sustainable Development Goals. Available at:* https://sdgs.un.org/2030agenda (accessed December 2022).

UN (2019) *World Population Prospects 2019: Highlights*. United Nations Department of Economic and Social Affairs, Population Division, ST/ESA/WER.A/423. Available at: https://population.un.org/wpp/publications/files/wpp2019_highlights.pdf (accessed December 2022).

UN-Habitat (2020) *World Cities Report: The Value of Sustainable Urbanization*. United Nations Human Settlements Programme. Available at: https://unhabitat.org/wcr (accessed June 2022).

Victor, D. (2015) Climate change: embed the social sciences in climate policy. *Nature* 520, 27–29. doi: 10.1038/520027a

Warwick, C. and Steedman, C. (2021) Wildlife-pet markets in a one-health context. *International Journal One Health* 7(1), 42–64.

WHO (2021) *Urban Health*. World Health Organization. Available at: www.who.int/news-room/fact-sheets/detail/urban-health (accessed June 2022).

WHO (2022) *Food Safety*. World Health Organization. Available at: www.who.int/news-room/fact-sheets/detail/food-safety (accessed June 2022).

The Human–Animal Bond

3

Carla Finzel[1]* and Jo Hockenhull[2]
[1]*District Veterinary Nurse, UK and founder of the DVN Hub;* [2]*University of Bristol, UK*

Key Points

- History of the human–animal bond (HAB)
- Physical and psychological benefits
- Specific population groups and HAB
- Animal-assisted interventions
- Facilitating a successful HAB

3.1   Brief History of the Human–Animal Bond

Humans have co-existed with a variety of animal species for thousands of years. Some species became domesticated under humans at different times and by different processes, depending on the species biology, human cultures and the opportunities presented (Zeder, 2012). Domestication enabled humans to control the location of the animals, how they were fed and how they were bred (Zeder, 2012). The outcome of this process impacts our lives today through the animals we eat and those we have in our homes. There are several key traits that predispose animals to domestication; typically, they are social species with a generalized diet and a straightforward reproductive strategy with low reactivity to people and sudden environmental changes (Price, 1984). Once domesticated, animals have served various roles, including protection, traction, clothing, transport, food, entertainment, sport and companionship. The role that each species plays in human lives may vary considerably over time, geographical location, culture and necessity, with many occupying several different roles within their human's environment.

   While there is evidence of individual close relationships between animals and people throughout history, pet ownership as we know it is a more recent

*Email: carla@dvnhub.com

© CAB International 2023. *One Health for Veterinary Nurses and Technicians*
(eds R. Jones and A. Jeffery)
DOI: 10.1079/9781789249477.0003

phenomenon developing in the 19th century. Prior to this it was primarily the nobility who kept animals purely for pleasure and companionship, as they were the only people who could afford to feed an additional mouth that did nothing to earn its keep. With the Victorians, pet-keeping became mainstream and associated services such as pet food manufacturing and breed societies also became established at this time. Selective breeding for aesthetic qualities gained popularity and generated a range of different breed types in common pet species such as dogs, cats and rabbits, as pet owners sought animals that were distinctive and different from the norm. Similarly, today we are seeing an explosion of increasingly exotic animal species kept as pets (Grant *et al.*, 2017) such as hedgehogs, snakes, spiders and sugar gliders as people continue to seek novelty in their animal companions.

There is evidence throughout human history of emotional attachment to animals, from ancient burials of humans with dogs with the bodies arranged to imply an affectionate relationship between the two, to the more modern pet graveyards and their enduring monuments to companionship lost through death. How companion animals are perceived by wider society has also changed over this time and these societal norms have implications for animal husbandry and management. For example, dogs have transitioned from being kept outside and fed on household scraps to living in the house, being fed bespoke food, and even sleeping in their owner's bed. Most pet owners consider their companion animal to be a member of their family, with all that entails in terms of home comforts and medical (veterinary) care, particularly if their pet is a cat or dog (Gates *et al.*, 2019). There is mounting evidence to suggest that the bonds formed between humans and their animal companions are similar to the attachment bonds formed between a human mother and infant. Much of this research has focused on dogs (Gácsi *et al.*, 2013), the first animal species domesticated, whose co-evolution with humans has led to an impressive ability to read and follow human behavioural cues, creating arguably the closest of human–animal relationships.

Alongside the change in views regarding companion animals, there have been corresponding changes in societal practices to cater for the human–animal bond within human activities. Companion animals can now be taken into cafés, go on public transport and even take holidays with their owners – provided that they stay in pet-friendly accommodation. Some workplaces allow people to bring their animal companions to work with them and there are calls for employers to allow staff to take compassionate leave when they lose a pet, due to the emotional toll this can have (SCAS, 2020). Growing societal recognition of the significance of animal companionship within human lives is testament to the value placed on these close bonds. It also demonstrates the way in which human practices and perceptions evolve over time, and the consequences this can have for the animals we share our lives with.

The COVID-19 pandemic provides a good example of how a change in human behaviour can impact pet ownership. From early 2020, mandatory UK government restrictions, imposed to control the spread of the virus, meant that people were encouraged to work from home where possible. The opportunities for in-person social interaction with people not in the same household were also significantly reduced during these lockdowns; non-essential shops were closed and social gatherings were banned. During this period there was a significant rise in pet ownership across multiple species. In the UK alone, 3.2 million household have acquired a pet since the pandemic began (PFMA, 2021). Rescue centres rehomed far more animals than average and the increased demand for puppies led to the phenomenon of the 'pandemic puppy'. Research by the Kennel Club suggested that this was driven by a desire for lockdown companionship (Kennel Club, 2020). The seismic shift in pet ownership during this period had consequences which are now being felt as COVID-19 restrictions have ended, and people are returning to their pre-COVID routines and behaviour patterns. In the Kennel Club study, 20% of respondents had not considered the long-term commitment they were making when they took on their puppy and had not thought about how they would manage when they returned to work.

Data from 2021 suggest that 17 million homes in the UK have pets, equating to 34 million animals, including 12 million dogs, 12 million cats, 3.2 million small mammals (such as rabbits, guinea pigs and hamsters), 3 million birds and 1.5 million reptiles (PFMA, 2021). This does not include fish, which are measured by tank or pond rather than individual numbers. The human desire for animal companionship is as great as ever and understanding what it is that people and animals get out of their interspecies relationships is the focus of the next section.

3.2   Physical and Psychological Benefits of the Human–Animal Bond

Companion animals, commonly known as pets, are not just cats and dogs. As per the data provided in section 3.1, many other species are included within this denomination. The bond that can develop between humans and their companion animals can greatly enrich the lives of both parties in a variety of ways, but it is important to recognize that there can also be downsides. Despite popular opinion suggesting that pet ownership has multiple physical and psychological benefits, the scientific evidence underlying this claim is not clear cut (McNicholas *et al.*, 2005; Gee and Mueller, 2019). Some of the research into this area has provided mixed results and while there is evidence that pet ownership can improve mental and physical health, interpreting these findings is not always straightforward, due to potential confounding factors. For example, is it owning a dog or the extra exercise that comes with dog ownership that provides the benefit? Often, we see a publication bias towards the studies that have found evidence of positive benefits of pet ownership; these are the studies that are typically picked up by the mainstream press rather than those that found no effect of pet ownership at all. This so-called 'halo effect', which implies that health improvements can be gained by merely acquiring a pet (Scoresby *et al.*, 2021), must be recognized for what it is, to promote a more realistic, evidence-based view on the physical and psychological consequences of pet ownership.

That said, there is a growing body of evidence that does suggest that owning a pet can improve the health of the owner, including their cardiac health, physical fitness through increased exercise, mental health (for example, reducing symptoms of depression), reduced loneliness and increased social functioning in some populations (Gee and Mueller, 2019). Additionally, we know that simply being around animals can have a positive impact on mental wellbeing. The numerous human support activities that animals are a key part of, such as emotional support and therapy animals, are a testament to the benefits that their presence can have (see section 3.5: Assistance Animals). We need to acknowledge, however, that little is known about the effect these activities have on the animals involved (for example, see review by Glenk (2017) on therapy dog welfare).

In addition to the benefits of being around animals, having an animal in your life can provide a plethora of other advantages that positively impact human quality of life. Caring for a pet brings responsibility, routine and structure to life, something that is recognized as being particularly important for people with poor mental health, older people who otherwise live alone and homeless people. Pets provide companionship and social support and can make it easier to engage in social contact with other people; for example, being out with a dog can facilitate social interactions with other walkers. The strength of the human–animal bond not only has a beneficial effect at an individual level, physically and mentally, but it also improves health at a community level, contributing to social capital (McNicolas and Collis, 2000; Melson, 2002). Wood *et al.* (2007) described dog walking as social lubrication with contacts extending beyond the dog owners themselves to the residents in a community who were not themselves dog owners.

Zooeyia is a word used to describe the positive health benefits of pets to human beings (Noah and Ostrowski, 2018) and companion animals (pets) can be a valuable resource to general practitioner doctors (GPs) and other health providers, which may help their human patients take better care of themselves. One example could be smoking cessation, as it affects their animal companion inadvertently via passive smoking (see Chapter 4, Non-Communicable Diseases and Other Shared Health Risks).

Under the umbrella of One Health, the first author of this chapter [CF] would advocate human health general practitioners and human-centred nurses asking their patients if they live with an animal. This question not only opens communication but can help the health practitioner and the patient strengthen their relationship. An example is given in Box 3.1.

This is an example of how One Health could be championed: collaboration between the veterinary and human-centred teams within the community. All human–animal bonds could be supported through the building of trust, and the incorporation of the pets into the treatment plans of the owners needing

---

Box 3.1. Do you live with an animal?

I am worried about my health because I have searched the internet about my symptoms and have read advice that I should really speak with my doctor. However, I am concerned that if I speak to my doctor, it may lead to me needing to go into a hospital for further tests or procedures and I would be worried about what would happen to my dog. The uncertainty and distress of not knowing who would walk them or give them their daily medication might mean that I do not want to speak with my doctor. It would help if, during the consultation, I was asked:

- Do you share your life with a pet?
- What species is your pet?
- Are you worried about them if you were to become unwell? Would you like us to have name and details of the veterinary practice that you are registered with?

---

care. People are so worried about what would happen to their beloved animal companions, in many instances their sole companions, if they needed to have a healthcare intervention that took them away from their home. Therefore, there need to be pathways to reassure the owner and try to keep them together with their pet. Incorporating systems to enhance and solidify collaborative networks between veterinary teams and local community and district healthcare teams is an example of One Health.

Zoonosis is the definition for diseases that are transmittable from animals to humans, while reverse zoonosis refers to human-to-animal transmission (see Chapter 5: Communicable Diseases). What better way to mitigate zoonotic risks than human healthcare practitioners working together with veterinary professionals, including veterinary nurses? What better way to reassure human health practitioners than to have a connection with a veterinary team including a veterinary nurse working within the community when, for example, they are concerned that a human patient who is immunosuppressed due to a treatment for cancer may be at risk from their pet? Also, if there is communication (with patient consent) from the GP informing the veterinary surgeon that their client is undergoing cancer treatment, the veterinary surgeon can be mindful of some treatments for the pet as well as providing guidance regarding looking after the pet without compromising the owner's health. They can also assist with signposting to the appropriate support services. If owners could talk about their pets without being scared that their pets would be removed from their lives because of their own medical condition, veterinary nurses could, as part of the veterinary team, support both the veterinary surgeon and the human healthcare practitioners in supporting and advocating the human–animal bond and putting it at the core of One Health.

As indicated earlier in this chapter, there is evidence of health improvements through pet ownership. Box 3.2 gives some expanded examples.

As discussed, pets were a common source of stress and concern for their owners during the COVID-19 pandemic as they worried about how they could

Box 3.2. Examples of health improvement through pet ownership.

Reduction of cardiovascular disease risks
This is mainly associated with dog ownership. The increased motivation to exercise and to lead a healthier lifestyle has a positive impact on the health of dog owners/caregivers (Levine *et al.*, 2013).

Alleviation of stress and anxiety
The interaction with a pet has the potential to induce feelings of relaxation and increasing one's sense of wellbeing (HABRI, 2022a).

Increase in self-esteem
Particularly for children and teenagers, caring for a pet will allow them to learn valuable lessons about responsibility and duty for their future adult life (Endenburg and van Lith, 2011).

Children on the autism spectrum and with other learning difficulties
A pet can act as a transitional aider, facilitating positive social interactions with family members. Additionally, the interaction with a pet can help to lower the child's stress and aid them to cope better when frustration sets in (HABRI, 2022b).

Companionship
When you have a pet, you might be alone, but you are rarely lonely (except when your cat goes for a three-day wander!) (Staats *et al.*, 2008).

Pet ownership increases sociability
Walking a dog, or conversing with other people about your beloved pet, encourages interaction with other members of the community, helping to form strong bonds and a stronger community sense (HABRI, 2022c).

care for them practically and financially, due to restricted access to shops and other resources at this time (Applebaum *et al.*, 2020). Life with an animal may not always go according to plan and there may be health or behavioural issues that require additional time, money and commitment to resolve. Unfortunately, the realities of life can make it difficult for some pet owners to commit to what their animal needs or keep their companion animal as long as they would have wished. For example, a change in personal circumstances can mean that someone may no longer have the ability to look after their animal as they once did. People in this situation can feel frightened of speaking about it through fear of being judged. As a veterinary nurse, providing non-judgemental guidance and support to these owners can help them through this challenging time and help them decide what is best for their pet.

The physical and psychological impacts of the human–animal bond for the animal are equally as mixed but altogether much less researched. Ideally pets should have their basic needs met at the very least, for example nutritious food, a safe environment and veterinary treatment, but through ignorance or intentional neglect this is not always the case. Some problems, such as obesity, may stem from a misdirected desire by the owner to demonstrate their love to their pet, without taking their pet's needs into account. The companionship provided by their owner can be a positive addition to the lives of some pet species, most notably dogs, who have co-evolved to live with people over thousands of years. However, for other species, such as rabbits and guinea pigs, a human companion cannot replace companionship of their own kind. We know that animals can be highly attuned to human behaviour, which is why they can make such valuable therapy and support animals, yet at present we do not know enough about how this may impact the animal.

It is important to recognize that no matter how much we love our companion animals and consider them family members, our relationship is not based on an equal footing. There is a power imbalance within any human–animal relationship, with the humans holding the power. The human caregiver typically determines what the animal is fed and when, where they can go, who they can socialize with, the veterinary treatment they receive and whether they can reproduce. This will vary to a greater or lesser extent depending on the species of animal, societal norms, personal attitudes and finances. By acknowledging the power imbalance within the human–animal bond we are also acknowledging the responsibilities we have towards the animals in our care. Rather than detracting from the emotional significance of these interspecies relationships, this acknowledgement can empower people to advocate on behalf of their companion animals.

Overall, the benefits for human wellbeing from sharing our lives with animals are thanks to the affection and comfort they provide via the human–animal bond. The human–animal bond has huge benefits for the humans; we just need to ensure that we advocate for the animal too, to ensure a mutual benefit of this bond.

3.3   Potential Implications of the Human–Animal Bond

The bond that humans have with their companion animals and their attitudes towards them can have serious implications for the health and welfare of the animal, the quality of the human–animal bond, and the benefits the human derives from it. There are several factors that may contribute to attitude formation and these will be discussed below, along with their consequences for the animal and the relationship between animal and human. It is often easier for a veterinary nurse to be objective about an animal's health and welfare than it is for their owner. While this can facilitate decision making from a veterinary perspective, it is important to understand the unique perspective of each owner and how this may influence their thought process when it come to the care their animal receives.

Anthropomorphism is the attribution of human characteristics, including emotions and behaviour, to non-human animals, objects and other entities. Most of us have grown up with the idea that animals possess human traits; after all, humanized animals are common subjects of children's books and movies. It may seem like harmless fun, but anthropomorphism can have serious implications for how we treat animals. By imbuing animals with human traits, we are overlooking much of what makes them animals and this can create a mismatch between our expectations and reality. For example, one consequence of overestimating the reasoning abilities of animals is to believe they perform unwanted behaviour on purpose, that they are deliberately scratching furniture or toileting in the house to make a point. There is no evidence that animals have these abilities, but if their human believes that they do, they may be tempted to punish the animal for their 'wrongdoing'. Such punishment would not be appropriate and can seriously harm the human–animal bond. Underestimating an animal's abilities can equally cause problems. Many people do not appreciate the sentience and cognitive abilities of animals and therefore see no harm in confining them in restricted and unstimulating environments. Others may not believe that animals experience pain, which may mean they do not seek veterinary treatment if their animal is unwell or injured. Unrealistic expectations within a human–animal relationship not only impact the way an animal may be treated but may also impact the owner. A person who feels that their animal is doing certain behaviours on purpose to spite them is not going to take pleasure from that relationship, no matter how much they love their companion. Should the situation continue there is a risk that the animal may be rehomed or relinquished to a rescue centre, which has implications for their welfare as well as negative consequences for the owner if they associate this decision with guilt or feelings of failure. Fortunately, there is a growing body of recognized behaviour professionals who can work with people and their animals to overcome these misunderstandings and help rebuild their relationships. Veterinary nurses are well placed to advise and to signpost owners in such circumstances to appropriate sources of support.

Anthropomorphism may lead people to make inappropriate choices when it comes to their animal's diet and environment too. By thinking that our animals will enjoy what we enjoy, we risk making management decisions that are inappropriate or even harmful. Providing animals with human food is one example of this, risking digestive upset, obesity or even poisoning. Most animals need time to roam freely and engage in species-specific behaviours. While a cage or hutch may look cosy and safe to us, it may not be perceived the same way by animals who use flight to escape things they are scared of. Some of our companion animals are highly social, for example guinea pigs and rabbits. While a person may feel they provide enough companionship for their animal, this is not the same as living with a conspecific; these animals need companionship of their own kind. Understanding and providing for the species-specific needs of companion animals will not only enhance their health and wellbeing but will also result in a human–animal bond that is based on knowledge rather than unrealistic expectations of the animal, ultimately leading to a more satisfying and less stressful relationship for both parties. These species-specific needs should be accommodated within veterinary practice as far as possible too. For example, bonded animals such as rabbits and guinea pigs can be brought in together for companionship and social support even if only one of them needs to see a vet. Veterinary nurses are well placed to advise on this.

Anthropomorphism is not all bad. In some situations, by putting ourselves into our animals' shoes we can better empathize with them and gain a better appreciation of how they experience different situations. During the COVID-19 pandemic many parallels were drawn between the experiences of humans during lockdown and the lived experiences of captive and domestic animals – including physical restrictions, social isolation, and loss of choice and control. Such comparisons triggered an empathetic response in some people who had not considered animal lives from that perspective before. Thinking about how they would feel in a given situation may help people make more considered choices for their animals regarding their management and welfare. However, it is critical that they remember that their animal is just that, an animal, and will have their own species-specific likes, dislikes and preferences in how they spend their lives.

Animals are individuals, each with unique personalities shaped by their genetics, environment, experiences and learned behaviour. This is not anthropomorphic. There is a large body of scientific literature documenting evidence of animal personality in a wide range of species, including amphibians, reptiles, fish, birds and mammals (Stamps and Groothuis, 2010; Wilson *et al.*, 2019). Getting to know an animal's personality is part of getting to know them as an individual and developing a close human–animal bond. Understanding an animal's personality will help predict how they will respond in different situations, enabling steps to be taken to manage these in the interests of the animal.

As discussed above, the decisions humans make often have immediate implications for their animals and potentially lasting consequences for both parties. There are two good examples of this.

Firstly, the phenomenon of COVID-19 pets, the upsurge in the acquisition of companion animals of all species as discussed above. Many people were first-time pet owners, and most took the opportunity they had of being at home all the time to get a new animal companion. Unfortunately, as the lockdowns ended and people started to return to working outside the home, they realized that they did not have the ability to take care of their new pet when real life resumed. There was an increase in animals being advertised online as needing to be rehomed as the owner could no longer give them the time they needed. For those animals who remained in their homes, other problems manifested such as separation anxiety in dogs as their owners were suddenly absent from the house for large parts of the day. This phenomenon had significant emotional implications for both humans and animals. Humans were forced to make difficult decisions regarding the feasibility of maintaining the human–animal bond they had sustained during lockdown, likely leading to feelings of guilt and loss. The animals were subject to dramatic changes in their home environment whether they stayed or were rehomed, and this was likely to be detrimental for their wellbeing.

The second example concerns end-of-life decision making. Deciding when it is time to euthanize a companion animal who is suffering is never easy. It is often the hardest decision people ever have to make and one that stays with them forever. The difficulty in saying goodbye can lead to euthanasia being delayed until the owner is ready to let go, potentially at the expense of the animal's welfare. Negotiating this issue can be challenging for all involved – owner, animal and veterinary team – but there are ways to facilitate this process, as discussed in section 3.6 below. It is important that these situations are approached with compassion. Letting go is difficult, but prolonging ineffective treatment and unnecessary suffering is wrong. Humanely ending the suffering of our animal companions is the last kindness that we can do for them. Recognizing how the human–animal bond can influence decision making in this context and the emotional impact this has on the human left behind can help veterinary nurses navigate this situation and support the human while helping them come to terms with what may be best for their animal.

3.4   Specific Groups and the Human–Animal Bond

People can experience having a pet at different stages in their lives. For some people, having a pet has been an integral part of their lives, growing up with them as a child, and enjoying the benefits of having a four-legged friend, whilst learning the responsibilities of caring for another living being at the same time. For others, pets come later in their life, for example when entering a life-partnership or marriage or a change in personal circumstances driving the individual to look for the companionship of a pet. In some cases, a pet is welcomed to complete the family unit by those who had a pet during their childhood and would like to replicate the experience for their own children. Less commonly, but just as importantly, a pet can enter someone's life as a therapy pet (for example, a dog, cat, rabbit, bird), becoming an essential part of that person's existence.

The Equality Act (2010) brought together over 116 separate pieces of legislation into one single Act. It provides a legal framework to protect the rights of individuals and advance equality of opportunity for all. One piece of legislation that has merged into this Act is The Disability Discrimination Act (1995) (Equality and Human Rights Commission, 2020).

There are about 13.3 million disabled people in the UK (almost one in five of the population); 17% of disabled people are born with a disability but most people acquire their disability later in life (Papworth Trust, 2018).

Types of disability that veterinary nurses should be aware of include:

- Physical disability
- Intellectual disability
- Communication disability
- Learning disability
- Sensory disability
- Mental health disability.

Box 3.3. Visible and non-visible disabilities.

Visible disabilities
When living with a physical disability (a visible disability), tasks like the examples listed below can prove challenging:

- Opening and closing doors
- Dressing and undressing
- Loading and emptying the washing machine
- Picking up items dropped, like keys or a bag
- Reaching up to the counter to pick up an item like a book or a mobile phone

(Source: Dogs for Good, available at: www.dogsforgood.org (accessed May 2022))

Non-visible disability
A non-visible disability is one that is not immediately obvious. Examples include:

- Health conditions such as diabetes and chronic pain
- Cognitive impairment such as dementia, autism and mental health conditions

Some more detailed examples are included below.

3.4.1 Aphasia

Aphasia is a communication disability which occurs when the communication centres of the brain are damaged. It is usually caused by a stroke, brain haemorrhage, head injury or a brain tumour. Aphasia makes it difficult to read, write or speak. It affects people differently: some people are unable to speak at all, others may have difficulty finding the right words to say or have difficulty reading, writing or using numbers. It affects relationships, employment, education, social lives and confidence. Aphasia affects around 350,000 people in the UK, yet not many people have heard of it. The fact that this condition is rarely heard of contributes to the loneliness that aphasia sufferers experience.

The human–animal bond between people living with aphasia and their animal companion is very strong and meaningful. These bonds prove invaluable in combating the isolation and loneliness that can be experienced through the barriers in communication with fellow humans. Animals do not speak our language, so automatically this barrier is non-existent and these are great friendships sustained by the ease and comfort provided in relationships with animals who are non-judgemental. Animals do not mind if we cannot talk, or write or read. They accept us as we are.

As veterinary nurses, we need to provide the tools to our pet owners so that they can communicate with us when their animals are unwell. Working with the charity Say Aphasia (www.sayaphasia.org), [CF] provides materials that help people with aphasia to communicate what they would like the veterinary nurse or surgeon to do with their animal.

3.4.2 Dementia

Veterinary nurses could be encouraged to become Dementia Friends. Dementia Friends is an Alzheimer's Society programme (Dementia Friends, 2022). A veterinary nurse who is a Dementia Friend is not an expert in dementia but is able to understand how a person living with dementia may perceive the world around them and most importantly can assist a pet owner with dementia in ensuring treatment care plans are carried out as prescribed by a veterinary surgeon. The veterinary nurse can help the veterinary surgeon to better communicate with the pet owner, and not to have expectations which they are unable to deliver. This enables the veterinary team to work effectively in facilitating a public service that adheres with the Equality Act of 2010.

3.4.3 Mental health

Pets undoubtedly offer companionship and affection to humans and the latter has been highlighted more than ever by the effects of the COVID-19 pandemic lockdown at an individual and societal level. Humans are a social species and social interaction is vital for our existence. Pets have proved to be an essential asset for families and individuals during the lockdown periods and their presence has been invaluable in helping to maintain the mental wellbeing of those who have been in isolation.

Mental health clinicians offer mindfulness as a tool for loneliness (Teoh *et al.*, 2021), encouraging the individual to become aware of their surroundings and to keep their mind focused on what is occurring at that present moment. In this task, pets can be a great help by encouraging their owners/caregivers to be in the present moment, and engaging them in play, walks, time outside or by merely stimulating their senses in a tactile way, such as when stroking their fur. For those of us blessed to share our lives with a pet, the COVID-19 lockdown periods enhanced the benefits of pet ownership on many levels, reducing isolation and offering us companionship, someone to talk to, physical connection and protection against loneliness. The realization of the benefits of pet ownership and the changes in work arrangements facilitated during lockdown has driven many people to consider welcoming a pet to their lives for the first time, particularly a dog, driving the boom in puppy ownership during lockdown. Loneliness is a risk factor for depression and anxiety symptoms. According to Bowen *et al.* (2021), the lockdown period caused an increase in depression and anxiety, particularly in single people and vulnerable people self-isolating, at a worldwide level. Using the pandemic as an example of how the human–animal bond alleviated the tough time of solitary confinement away from other people, Bowen *et al.* (2021) collected data from a selected population of Spanish dog owners and found that pet owners reported that their dogs were an invaluable source of companionship, providing a routine of regular physical activities and comfort.

Before the pandemic, we saw emerging within workplaces, such as offices, an encouragement for staff to bring their dogs to work and the phrase 'pet inclusivity' becoming a buzzword. When this phrase is seen in a job advertisement, it might be felt that an employer is more human or empathetic – that the employer understands and sees the world from a wider perspective and that perhaps their ethos and values are more compassionate. The aims behind creating a 'pet-inclusive' office space might include the following.

- **Reduction of stress.** Animals have a way of helping our brains produce serotonin and dopamine, just by having a cat or a dog around the office who brings a toy and nudges to play for a couple of minutes. This is so positive for mental wellbeing.
- **Collaboration.** If, say, another employee is quite shy and finds it tricky to interact with co-workers, a pet can start up conversations that are not just work related but more open ended and bring glimpses of a colleague's personality as they relax engaging in conversation. This may spark creativity and ignite the development of projects that are work related.
- **Job retention and recruitment.** Animals bring us joy and when we are happy we are more passionate, committed and invested in the things that make our life. Work is part of our lives. If a company promotes pet inclusivity, it may be more likely to understand and promote work/life balance, the importance of breaks to eat and rest. As we pause to consider the pet's needs, we may consider our own: take a lunchbreak, eat, go out in the fresh air for a 20-minute walk, for instance. Even people with no pets of their own tend to benefit from this. Some may wish they had a pet but maybe their circumstances prevent them from having an animal companion of their own, but coming to work and maybe sharing a lunchbreak dog walk with a co-worker who brings their dog to work could be so beneficial for their physical health and mental health.

The skillset of a veterinary nurse could be invaluable in helping companies to implement pet policies to ensure the welfare of the animals, because when pets are healthy, they are happy, and everyone benefits. The emotional wellbeing of the animals as well as their physical needs must be considered. If we look at the workplace policy from a veterinary perspective, it would be important to ensure that it states that an animal coming to the workplace should be neutered, up to date with preventive healthcare and free from disease. Behaviourally, for example, the animal should not be anxious or fearful of other pets and people and it should be assessed to determine its suitability to come into the workplace. Many people might assume that panting, for example, is due to the dog being hot, but a dog panting in a cool office could be exhibiting signs of stress. A veterinary nurse could raise awareness and suggest that a certified behaviourist, under veterinary referral, could be engaged by the company or employer. Any workplace assessment prior to pets entering would need to consider the safety of the office environment: what hazards there are, from an animal perspective, including electric wires, food in bags at ground level and toxic plants. There should also be consideration for the welfare of the animal, for example making sure that they have a safe space where they can get away from interactions and how to deal with multiple animals in the same office. All these factors could be assessed by a veterinary nurse working as part of the wider veterinary team

3.4.4 Homelessness

The human–animal bond between a homeless person and their animal companion can be very strong. For a homeless person and their animal companion, this relationship can provide benefits such as safety and emotional support (Kerman *et al.*, 2019) at a time when the homeless person can feel vulnerable and alone. Many homeless people will turn down a bed overnight in a hostel if their animal companion is not allowed in the premises. In this respect, the relationship faces challenges where both the pet and the human have decreased access to accommodation. One of the aims of the outreach organization, StreetVet, is to support hostels with the implementation of positive pet policies through their accredited hostel scheme (StreetVet, 2022). This is also a challenge faced by people who have a pet and are not considered homeless. The UK rental market is restrictive in allowing pets in rented accommodation.

In the USA, the Pet-Inclusive Housing Initiative conducted by Michelson Found Animals in collaboration with the Human Animal Bond Research Institute (HABRI) set out to tackle misconceptions about pets in rental housing (HABRI, 2022d). It revealed that not all 'pet-friendly' policies meant all pets were welcome. In some instances, there were restrictions on breeds and size. It challenged that these restrictions are not necessary, as owners of both pet-friendly accommodation and non-pet-friendly accommodation believe that adults and children were more likely to cause damages than cats or dogs, with only 9% of pets causing damage and 75% of residents preferred to live next door to a family that had pets than to adults in the college-student age group. The overall outcome was that 71% of residents agreed that pets bring the community together and 93% of both pet owners and property providers agreed that pets are important family members. Perhaps we need to see this shift in the UK.

3.4.5 Understanding disabilities

Whilst not working outside their legal remit and working alongside human healthcare providers, the veterinary nurse can adjust the method of veterinary nursing treatment care plan delivery (as directed by the veterinary surgeon) to best suit the medical conditions the pet owners live with through an understanding of their challenges. An owner may prefer factual and concise communication rather than a wordy information sheet. For example: 'Felix needs to have one eye drop in each eye, 4 times a day, which is every 6 hours. We have this tick chart to help you keep track, with days and times printed on it, you tick the boxes relevant to the day and time you administer the eye drops.'

Inclusion of disabled people into everyday activities involves practices and policies designed to remove barriers, whether physical, communication or attitudinal, that can affect an individual's ability to have full participation in society in the same way as people without disability. Inclusion involves fair treatment from others, making products, communications and the physical environment more usable and accessible for all.

Animals can help to eliminate the belief that people with disabilities are less capable of being integrated. These meaningful, animal-interactive companionships can make a difference for a person living with disabilities, whether visible or non-visible. However, when their animal becomes unwell, it can be a devastating and emotional situation for their human–animal bond. Sometimes, a person living with a disability cannot administer the treatment care plans as prescribed by the veterinary surgeon caring for the animal, resulting in separation: the animal may need to be hospitalized or placed in kennels to receive the treatment care plan. The animal may become depressed away from the human they assist, as this is their purpose, focus and their way of life, while their human is left without their most vital companion. A veterinary nurse working within the community could remove some of the barriers to disabled people caring for their pets, in line with the inclusion principle.

3.5　Animal-Assisted Interventions

3.5.1　Terminology

It is important to begin this section with three key terms related to this topic.

- **Human–animal bond (HAB):** a mutually beneficial and dynamic relationship between people and animals that is influenced by behaviours that are essential to the health and wellbeing of both.
- **Human–animal interactions (HAI):** the emotional, psychological and physical interactions of people, animals and the environment.
- **Animal-assisted interventions (AAI):** purpose-integrated and organized interventions that intentionally bring animals together with health, education and human service settings, with the objective to gain therapeutic benefits for better human health – physical and mental wellness (Pet Partners, 2019).

Animal-assisted interventions (AAI) is an umbrella term that describes any work with a therapy animal and includes:

- Animal-assisted therapy (**AAT**)
- Animal-assisted education (**AAE**)
- Animal-assisted activities (**AAA**).

Some key AAI definitions are set out in Table 3.1.

Whether a therapy animal is participating in AAT, AAE or AAA often depends on the qualifications of the handler and the goal of the visit.

- If a therapy animal is working with a professional to meet a client's formal treatment plan, they are engaged in AAT. An example might be therapeutic horse riding for autistic children (Learning Disability Today, 2022).
- Similarly, if a therapy animal is brought into an educational plan to meet formal objectives as measured by a professional, it is AAE. An example is the HABRI Listening Ears programme (HABRI, 2022e).
- Finally, there are therapy animal handlers who work as volunteers in the UK and the USA. These people give their time to go with their therapy animals to places such as hospitals, prisons and residential treatment facilities, to share the love of their pets. This is AAA. Further recommended reading can be found at the end of the chapter.

3.5.2 History of therapy animals

The history of therapy dogs and their beneficial influence in stress management disasters indicates that, in ancient times, the Egyptians, Greeks and Romans recognized that animals provided therapy to humans. In the 18th century in York, England, William Tuke raised funds to open the York Retreat for people with mental 'illness', as it was called in those days; he recognized that small animals, which freely inhabited the grounds of the York Retreat, had a therapeutic effect.

In the 19th century, animals supported the treatment of people at Bethel, a residential facility in Germany for young people with epilepsy. During the Crimean War, Florence Nightingale recommended that cats should be kept as companions for the chronically ill, as well as for rat control (Shubert, 2012).

Table 3.1. Key definitions in animal-assisted interventions (based on definitions from Pet Partners, 2019)

Term	Definition
Handler	The person who owns the therapy animal and goes with the therapy animal to the facility.
Therapy animal	The animal who *willingly* participates in the animal-assisted intervention.
Client	The human who benefits from the animal-assisted intervention.
Facility	The place where the animal-assisted intervention takes place and where the handler and the therapy animal meet the client. This may be, for example, a hospital, a school, a prison, a care home, a crisis scene like a mountain rescue.

3.5.3   Understanding therapy and assistance animals

Animal-assisted interventions are becoming more widely known, including for people whose lives become brighter when visited by a therapy animal and the impact they can have, such as within education. One such example was provided by the Human Animal Bond Research Institute (HABRI, 2022e) when third-grade students in the USA, who were struggling to read, had therapy rabbits visiting the school. The research demonstrated that the students lost inhibition and found it easier to read when reading to a rabbit.

HABRI (2022c) also reports how people become more independent when an assistance animal lives with them. Sharing life with an assistance animal can be invaluable to gain emotional confidence and feel integrated in society, for example going out shopping with an assistance animal that has been trained to retrieve items on the shop shelves that are out of reach. Meeting people and chatting opens a whole world of possibilities, which is good for our mental health.

When veterinary nurses provide care to patients who are assistance animals, they need to:

- recognize the importance of their role in maintaining and promoting animal welfare;
- be aware of the ethics framework of animal-assisted interventions; and
- be aware of the working protocols as laid out in the Standards of Practice of Animal-Assisted Interventions (Pet Partners, 2019) (see section 3.5.7 below).

Whether the animal is a visiting therapy animal who belongs to a handler or a therapy animal who lives with a pet owner with non-visible or visible disability, the veterinary nurse is pivotal in raising awareness of the welfare of their patients. When there is a concern that a patient's welfare is compromised in any way it, is important to flag to the veterinary surgeon so that an assessment can be made regarding the patient's welfare. If necessary, it may be that the veterinary nurse or veterinary surgeon contact the organization which provides the animal-assisted intervention.

It is recommended that veterinary nurses are equipped with knowledge of the Standards of Practice of Animal-Assisted Interventions when caring for assistance animals, as this will support them in recognizing whether the handler, pet owner or organization is promoting animal welfare, maintaining the ethics of their professions so as to best support each other in providing well managed and safe interactions, where both animals and humans are happy and can thrive.

The veterinary nurse needs to understand the specific training which enables animals to qualify as a therapy or assistance animal and the specific needs that they have.

When the needs of these animals are optimally met, it means that they will not be subjected to work they cannot perform and, when they are unwell, these animals, who are used to working, can still have a stimulated recovery time. For example, if a dog cannot work as a guide dog due to lameness, the veterinary nurse can work with the owner to determine if the patient can instead be mentally stimulated by doing some gentle scent work at home.

One example in terms of understanding the role of an assistance animal would be the dog of a person living with Ehlers Danlos syndrome. According to the Ehlers Danlos Organization in the UK: *'Ehlers Danlos Syndromes (EDS) are a group of thirteen individual genetic conditions affecting the body's connective tissue. People with EDS tend to experience a broad range of symptoms, including long-term pain, chronic fatigue, dizziness, dislocations, and digestive disorders.'*

An assistance animal may assist the human with picking up things that drop on the floor, whatever they may be, so even if someone puts a crumpled piece of paper in the bin, the dog could recognize it as a fallen item and return it to the person that dropped it. In this case, it may be the veterinary nurse who, whilst visiting the patient and owner in their home to administer medication to the dog, has put the piece of paper in the bin. When assisting a pet owner with Ehlers Danlos syndrome, the veterinary nurse will need to understand what an assistance animal has been trained to do and may need to refrain from doing certain things to prevent confusing their patient, including those activities that they may normally do without thinking. In the eyes of the assistance animal trained to fetch an item for a human with a condition that compromises their hand grip, causing items to be dropped unintentionally, this is a very important task and one which they might do several times in one day. If not rewarded for the action, or if the veterinary nurse drops it in the paper waste bin again, the dog may be confused, and even upset if the veterinary nurse's body language and reaction are not appreciative of their work.

3.5.4   The needs of therapy and assistance animals

We will now explore the needs of therapy animals and assistance animals and the thought that if they are 'workers', they have rights. If the animal is not registered with a recognized AAI organization, properly assessed to ensure that their physical and mental health are suitable for them to fulfil their roles safely and ensure their needs are met, then the five welfare needs (PDSA, 2022) are not being adhered to. The veterinary nurse, under veterinary direction, may be able to assess the following:

1. Behaviour – is the therapy animal enjoying the interaction and do they have a choice? Is performing this job suppressing natural behaviour all the time, or even any of the time? How are the rights of this therapy animal being observed (like any human worker); for example, how many hours is the animal required to work?
2. Environment – which ties in with the behaviour.
3. Diet – are they being fed the species-specific diet as per veterinary surgeon recommendation?

4. Companionship – company of their own kind if they enjoy the company of others, without aggression and stress, for emotional enrichment.

5. Health – preventive healthcare, treated appropriately for pain, disease and suffering.

3.5.5   Emotional support animals (ESA)

There is a distinct awareness that our beloved animal companions offer incredible emotional support just by sharing life with us. There is no doubt that, for example, heading to the stables to the horse after a busy day at work dealing with many deadlines can be so 'therapeutic' and grounding. We may go for a trek on the horse and look at a beautiful sunset, come back and, as we brush our horse, as we ensure the bedding is dry and thick for the night, as we provide fresh water and food, we somehow forget for a while the stress of the day, and everything feels all right. So, in that sense, our horse is a 'therapy animal assisting in our wellbeing' and indeed it is our reciprocal desire to ensure the wellbeing of our horse, providing their welfare needs.

Emotional support animals (ESA) are different from therapy animals and assistance animals. In North America, an emotional support animal is one whose primary role is to support one individual and is able (due to its role) to live in a household with a 'no pets' policy (Pet Partners, 2019).

Unlike in America, emotional support animals are not currently recognized as certified assistance animals in the UK. This means that the rules that apply to other assistance animals, such as guide dogs, do not apply to emotional support animals.

An organization does exist in the UK called the Emotional Support Animal UK registry, which was set up in 2017 to support those with emotional support animals by keeping a register of these animals and to lobby the UK government for a change in the legislation to include this group of support animals. Its website (ESA, 2022) states that: '*All domesticated animals may qualify as Emotional Support Animals and they can be any age, as these animals do not need any specific task-training like a service/assistance animal because their very presence alleviates the symptoms associated with a personal psychological or emotional disability.*'

3.5.6   Animal-assisted crisis response (AACR)

Another classification of assistance animal that is recognized in North America but not in the UK is that of animal-assisted crisis response.

According to Pet Partners (2019): '*AACR is a form of animal-assisted activities (AAA) that provides comfort to those who have been affected by natural, human-caused, or technological disasters. AACR is effective because the safety, familiarity, novelty, and interest in the animal have been found to be impactful when building rapport with a person affected by crisis.*'

AACR is not a professional mental health intervention. Pet Partners AACR handlers must complete online training, which includes psychological first aid concepts, sometimes also referred to as mental health first aid. This training has been designed with input from subject matter experts in the field.

AACR does not take the place of professional interventions but provides support in the immediate wake of a crisis through listening, empathy, and sharing the unconditional love of a therapy animal. AACR can be effective for everyone affected by the impact of a crisis, including first responders and crisis management staff.

There is a second organization in the USA called HOPE, which was also set up to provide emotional support to people (HOPE Animal-Assisted Crisis Response, 2022), and they describe the settings where their dogs and handlers provide animal-assistance crisis response:

- Death notifications
- Traumatic incidents that affect a school student body
- Suicides, accidental deaths, line-of-duty deaths
- Structure fires and Wildfire Base Camps
- Multi-casualty incidents
- Emergency rooms, ICU waiting areas following major incidents
- Emergency simulation drills
- Assisting behavioural health staff
- For pastoral services at hospitals, fire departments, law enforcement agencies, and congregations following major incidents
- Memorial services

3.5.7   Standards of Practice in Animal-Assisted Interventions

Whether the veterinary nurse works in the UK, in the USA, or anywhere else in the world, they can have a role, alongside veterinary surgeons, in supporting with treatment plans and nursing care of animals who have an assistance role. Handlers and pet owners are unlikely to be qualified veterinary professionals and it is vital to work in collaboration with the handlers/owners and the therapy animal's or assistance animal's veterinary surgeon, as well as any human health care organizations, to ensure a holistic approach to the care of both animal and human.

[CF] advocates the Standards of Practice in Animal-Assisted Interventions (Pet Partners, 2019) which is used as a guide to her own veterinary nursing practice as an advocate of assistance animal welfare. The Standards of Practice in Animal-Assisted Interventions lay out the safety of assistance and therapy animals, handlers and clients (the humans they are assisting).

The guidelines within the Standards are based on the belief that animals are not tools but sentient beings, that conditions must allow them to make choices and always express themselves and want to partake in an activity, and to ensure that the animals are protected and not exploited.

The Standards of Practice are a source of reference to incorporate best practices, whether the animal-assisted intervention is to be provided for a facility, individuals or organizations. The goals are to provide consistency and structure, educational resources for personnel and staff, the health, welfare and safety of all involved (animal, handler and client), assess risks and quality of the activity and provide high quality of service to all clients.

Within the UK, in 2019 the Royal College of Nursing (RCN) published a protocol to support those in health care and allied health care environments who work with dogs in these settings (RCN, 2019.)

3.6   Facilitating a Successful Human–Animal Bond

Like any other successful relationship, maintaining a mutually enjoyable and beneficial human–animal bond does not happen by chance but needs ongoing commitment. One important element is trust. To maintain trust, behaviour needs to be predictable and consistent. This way the animal knows what to expect from their human in each situation, and what is expected from them. Equally the human can predict how the animal may react and shape their behaviour and expectations accordingly. Therefore, getting to know each other as individuals is so important for both humans and animals. Once you have an idea of what the other party likes and dislikes, fears and enjoys, you can make your relationship as positive as possible by doing more of the good stuff together and take decisions that avoid the bad stuff, or at least minimize exposure to it as far as possible.

Unfortunately, sometimes we must put our animals into situations that we know they will not enjoy, or perhaps may even fear. This is often what happens when it comes to veterinary visits. Being aware of how an animal may react in this situation through discussions with the owner allows you to plan and prepare for it. One way in which veterinary nurses can support this is by encouraging owners to come into the practice regularly with their animals to get them used to the veterinary practice environment. Some practices even offer free support sessions so that owners can work with a member of the practice staff to help their animal become more comfortable in these surroundings. Regularly visiting the vet in this way to simply 'hang out' and eat nice treats in the waiting room will reduce the association the animal has with vet visits and uncomfortable or painful procedures such as vaccinations. While visiting the vet's may not ever become an animal's favourite activity, with a little preparation it can at least become less stressful for the animal, their human and the practice staff.

A big part of getting to know each other is knowing what is normal for an animal as an individual. What are their habits? When do they make noises? Do these noises differ in different situations? How and where do they like to rest? By knowing what is normal, it is easier to recognize when something is wrong. Many owners do not recognize the significance of small changes in their animal's behaviour, but by asking the right questions, veterinary nurses can draw out any observations that owners may not have considered mentioning. Animals are often better at noticing these small behavioural changes than humans, with many being quick to spot when their human is acting differently from normal. It is this high level of attunement to human behaviour that makes some owners think that their companion animal can read their mind by knowing when they are in a hurry, going on holiday or about to take them to the vet. This ability, alongside changes in odour, is also responsible for the capabilities of animals, particularly dogs, to detect cancer or other health concerns such as oncoming epileptic fit, hypoglycaemia or a panic attack in their owners.

There is a growing body of professionals who can work with people and their animals to resolve any problems that may arise in a human–animal relationship. Knowing when external expert help may be needed and who to approach is important and is something that many people struggle with. It can be hard to navigate the ever-increasing number of industry bodies and changing terminology surrounding companion animal-related services for those seeking help with their animal companion. Directing people to a recognized, accredited organization is critical to ensure that any individual or organization has the necessary skills, experience, qualifications and training to provide evidence-based best practice that puts animal welfare first, and veterinary nurses are well placed to do this.

Greater emphasis is now being given to monitoring an animal's quality of life throughout their lifetime, rather than something that is done once an animal's health begins to deteriorate. This is an incredibly positive step forward, as it shows the value of really getting to know your animal as an individual and using that knowledge to evaluate their health and wellbeing on a continual basis. It can be very difficult to monitor our own animals objectively. Luckily, there are several different tools available that owners can be directed to, many developed by animal charities and freely available on their websites. These tools differ in the details but essentially provide a structure to help people apply their knowledge of their animal to routinely assess their wellbeing. This information can then be used to inform treatment plans, to evaluate the impact of any routine, medication, or management changes, as well as help with end-of-life decision making. By thinking more proactively about a companion animal's health and wellbeing throughout their lifetime, any changes that occur are likely to be recognized sooner than they otherwise might have been. Therefore, if remedial action is needed, it can be implemented earlier, when it is more likely to be effective.

3.6.1 Support for an ageing animal

Like humans, animals may need increasing support as they age and possibly environmental adaptations. Dietary changes or medications may also become necessary. Exercise requirements and abilities may change, for example dogs may need shorter, slower walks. There are steps that can be taken to ease this process in both animals and their people, and a veterinary nurse with an awareness of these can help to guide owners in making life easier for themselves and their animals when changes need to be made. People may have assistance aids such as handrails and stairlifts fitted to their home. They may need extra help to look after their animals, such as using a dog walker to take their companion out for a walk if they can no longer manage, or someone to clean out their smaller animals if it becomes too much. Both humans and animals alike may benefit from environmental changes, including the addition of non-slip coverings to slippery floors and installing ramps if stairs are too challenging. Animals may also benefit from the provision of additional steps or platforms to help them access higher areas such as sofas or beds if jumping up has become difficult. What is important to remember for both humans and animals is that there are plenty of freely available resources that can provide information and ideas for how to make life easier during the ageing process. There are also many sources of guidance and practical support, such as the Cinnamon Trust in the UK who help elderly and terminally ill people look after their animals so that they can remain together. Some charities provide credit-card sized cards saying that, if something happens to the person, their animals are home alone and will require assistance. The card can be filled out with the relevant details of who should be contacted to take care of them should the person be incapacitated. Other charities provide a service whereby people can register their animal so that, should anything happen to them, their animal will be taken care of by the charity. This process can help people overcome anxieties around their animal's future at what is already a difficult time. These initiatives demonstrate the value of having a plan in place should the worst happen to a human or their animal companion. Many owners are unaware that many of these initiatives exist, and veterinary nurses play an important role in signposting owners to potential sources of help and advice.

3.6.2 End of life for a companion animal

Thinking about the end of a companion animal's life is always hard at any time. However, if it comes to the moment that a decision must be made and no thought has been given to how someone wants to say goodbye to their companion, it can be incredibly difficult for them to process the options and to make a choice that they will be comfortable with in the future. It can be tempting to put off thinking about losing a companion, but we need to acknowledge that euthanasia is not just linked to old age and may be needed at any stage of an animal's life if they are suffering. End-of-life planning is increasingly gaining traction within a veterinary context. Discussing the options with a vet in advance and spending the time to think about what would be best for both human and animal, means that important decisions do not have to be made without preparation when emotions are already running high. Factors to consider include whether euthanasia will take place at home or the vet practice, what should happen to the remains and whether the owner would like any type of memento such as a paw print or some hair to be taken. Different options may be available for different species and at different vet practices, so for veterinary nurses, knowing what is available in a particular scenario is important. Obviously, life does not always go according to plan and sometimes circumstances mean that an end-of-life plan cannot be followed exactly. But at least by having already considered the options and discussed the practicalities with the veterinary team, the owner will not be caught off-guard when the time comes.

The loss of a companion and subsequent end of a human–animal bond can be extremely distressing for both the human and the animal. As companion animals are being increasingly viewed as family members, the devastation caused by their loss is becoming more widely acknowledged within society. There is growing support available to people who have had to say goodbye to their animal companion. For example, the Blue Cross (2022) provides a free-of-charge Pet Bereavement Support Service where support can be sought by phone, email, live web chat or social media. There is also a growing number of counsellors who specifically offer services surrounding pet bereavement. A key consideration in this process is the role that guilt may play. Unlike typical human bereavement, grief is often compounded by guilt and regret in companion animal owners who have had to actively take the decision to end their animal's life. When to make the decision is highly subjective and will depend on an individual's beliefs, perceptions and circumstances. It is not uncommon for people to receive unhelpful comments from others about the animal being euthanized too early when they could have had more time together or too late when they were already suffering. Helping people come to terms with the decision they have taken is likely to be a big part of their grieving process.

It is important to recognize that grief may also impact animals left behind after the loss of their human companion, or indeed the loss of another animal companion. While discussions of animal grief have previously relied on anecdotal evidence (Bekoff, 2000), scientists are starting to explore this area in a more systematic way (Uccheddu *et al.*, 2022). Grief in animals manifests itself in a similar way to that in humans, with individuals becoming apathetic, depressed and losing their appetite (Uccheddu *et al.*, 2022). Animals who have lost their human typically experience a lot of change at this time, as they may be taken into the care of another person or organization, losing their familiar environment and routine as well as their caregiver. Compassion and understanding will be needed to help an animal through this time of upheaval. Often people have more than one companion animal. These may be separated after the loss of their human, adding another layer to their grief. It is equally important to recognize that animals may be affected by the death of another animal within their household. Navigating this experience with an animal that has been bereaved can be challenging for people if they too are mourning their missing animal companion. Giving the remaining animal the opportunity to inspect the body may help them to process the absence of their friend; however, it is critical that human observers do not expect human-like displays of grief from such an encounter. Such misplaced expectations may lead to anger if the animal is not seen to be expressing an 'appropriate' level of grief. Having open discussions around grief and bereavement with veterinary nurses can be beneficial for owners; however, it is important to ensure that the nurses themselves receive support and that the veterinary practice has appropriate training available and procedures in place to identify and reduce compassion fatigue within practice staff.

3.7 Caregiver Burden

Caregiver burden is defined as the level of multifaceted strain perceived by the caregiver from caring for a family member and/or loved one over time (Liu *et al.*, 2020).

The caregiver burden can be very real for pet owners. As a veterinary nurse it is one thing putting together a nursing care plan when you are writing this to be followed by fellow professionals but another thing when you are expecting it to be followed by pet owners, without the experience and competencies of a qualified veterinary nurse, to continue with the care plan as instructed when the patient is discharged. Animals are discharged with many complex treatment plans, for example feeding tubes, bandages, subcutaneous fluid administration, eye drop administration every two hours.

There needs to be a greater awareness and understanding of caregiver burden so that it can become an integral consideration when devising treatment care plans if we wish to achieve successful patient outcomes. The vet team–patient–pet owner relationship needs to be built on empathy and appreciation of the challenges pet owners face nursing our patients beyond the confines of the consulting rooms. When our clients experience our empathetic responses to these challenges, we can facilitate a psychological safe space where they can share their concerns regarding the treatment care plan. We can then work together to devise strategies that can help to alleviate the caregiver burden. Many pet owners are worried that they may be judged when feeding back to the veterinary surgeon about how they find their pet is progressing, and feel guilty at their inability to follow the steps of the treatment care plan. It is not that they were 'not compliant'; the reality is that they just struggled, as they are not veterinary professionals. A veterinary nurse can be instrumental in empowering pet owners and helping them gain a sense of control and self-esteem whilst adjusting their lives to caring for their animal companion during a convalescing period until they get better, or during a chronic condition or terminal disease.

Over seven years of practising as a veterinary nurse in the community, [CF] has collated a number of observations while working with pet owners nursing their pets at home:

- When we see a burdened caregiver, often the burden is constant problem solving, because new problems are always emerging when caring for a sick animal.
- The owner is constantly trying to decide whether the pet is getting worse or getting better, and they often do not have anyone to talk to about it, often leading to feelings of anxiety, constant vigilance and a potential sense of isolation and guilt.
- They can feel depression and anxiety as they are not supported in the care of their pet as they would be as human caregivers. 'My boss says, "It is just a dog", therefore is not going to give me time off work to take him to the vets, unlike giving my co-worker time off work to take her child to the doctor.'
- They can become exhausted and mental health/wellbeing can become compromised.

Now, consider when our clients are not equipped with the qualifications that we have and our professional skillset to implement veterinary nursing treatments:

- What questions are we asking the owners?
- Are we actively listening to their answers and doing the best we can to help them?
- Do we know anything about the owner's situation?
- Are owners able to communicate effectively with us and the vet?
- Are they truthful about their situation and home environment? Are they worried they will be judged and considered not competent?
- How many patients do we send home without truly knowing?
- Could we be doing more?

If a veterinary nurse is not available to outreach in the community, what can a veterinary nurse in practice do? We can actively listen to the pet owner and incorporate questions that can help the owner to feel safe to disclose if they are struggling. Sometimes, aside from any physical disability that may be a visible factor, we may find that there are non-visible disabilities that form part of the equation. Are the instructions given in a way that the owner/caregiver can find easy to understand and deliver? What may be considered easy to us may not be to them. It is important to explore with the owner what they feel would be most helpful rather than assume, but, as an example, written instructions may be preferable as verbal communication can be difficult to take onboard, especially when stressed or distracted.

We should listen to how the owners/caregivers are telling us their human–animal bond is being affected. Statements like when they report that their beloved animal companions may be 'weary' of them, listen to the cues when they say: 'Oh he just runs away when he sees me coming with the bottle of ear treatment, he just hates me now, he won't come in the house until we have gone to bed, and he was such a cuddly boy before, I just want him to like me again.'

Our role is to reassure the owner that the human–animal bond is not broken and that we are always here to chat if they are struggling; we can work together to try to find a solution, but advising them not to stop administering the treatment without sharing these challenges with us. It is important that we try not to get frustrated with the owner/caregiver and consider how we would like to be treated if it were us having this worry. Empathy and kindness are about 'I am here, and I am listening to your experience, and I am not judging you.'

It is important to remember we are all a team: the veterinary surgeon, the veterinary nurse and the owner/caregiver. At the core is the patient, who may be viewed as a family member. We all want for this animal to live well with the condition that has been diagnosed and for treatment care plans to work. However, there is no point expecting figs from an apple tree and labelling the apple tree 'non-compliant' if it cannot produce what it is not capable of. So, if the pet owner and veterinary nurse are part of the same team, we as the veterinary nurse within this team need to find the points of strength that we can work together with in putting together a care plan that works. Leadership is about finding the best in the people in our team and promoting their self-esteem. There is not 'them and us' in thriving teams so we should not treat the owner as 'them'. As veterinary nurses, we may also have animals ourselves and this can be a great bonding tool; it makes us more human and relatable, if we can share the challenges we have experienced with our own animals.

Working as a veterinary nurse in the community, this is what concordance means. It is about the pet owner and the veterinary team working together, with everyone understanding the need for the treatment care plan and working together to make it happen. Veterinary nursing in this setting is about facilitating client concordance. Concordance is the shared understanding between all participants and the veterinary nurse can play a key role in being that link between the veterinary surgeon and pet owner/caregiver.

In human healthcare, concordance is not synonymous with either compliance or adherence. Concordance does not refer to a patient's medicine-taking behaviour, but rather the nature of the interaction between clinician and caregiver, and their agreement (Brack et al., 2013). Every person is different. Generalizations and assumptions that all owners can and do assimilate instructions in the same way or can cope the same way leads to missed opportunities to generate concordance. Adaptations need to be considered for each owner when devising a treatment care plan.

Aligned with caregiver burden is compassion fatigue in veterinary professionals. All involved in the care of animals, and people, encounter compassion fatigue which is inevitable when working in close proximity to situations where, by the very nature of 'being caring' and doing the jobs that they do, they take on the feelings of others, like frustration at not being able to carry out a task, or grief for having lost a beloved animal companion. Compassion fatigue occurs when, in extending compassion to others, we do not allow a gap to reflect and think and process our own feelings and so are not able to recognize and talk about them (Cocker and Joss, 2016).

3.8   Summary

The impact of veterinary nurses and their work in the community is pivotal in supporting animal welfare. For many years human-centred nursing has had both community and district roles to support patients. This type of role is now developing within the veterinary nursing profession. Veterinary nursing in the community champions the power of animal companionship: the human–animal bond. This type of role has developed an innovative approach to supporting clients who are experiencing difficult times and protecting these meaningful bonds. As previously referenced, there is a wealth of evidence to demonstrate that a positive relationship between humans and animals can have a significant impact on human mental, emotional and physical health. Alongside the physical benefits, pet ownership can be particularly beneficial for those suffering from social isolation and/or mental health issues.

There are times when additional pressures in a person's life such as illness, financial crisis and homelessness can compromise the care of a beloved pet. In circumstances such as these, our skills as veterinary nurses alongside other veterinary and human healthcare professionals can bring the change needed and champion One Health.

All human–animal bonds need to be included so that these animals and humans do not fall through the cracks of society. There are many animals and pet owners that we do not get to see in our consulting rooms at our veterinary practices, through no fault of their own, and we must be proactive in putting systems in place to find and support them through work with charities like StreetVet and their 'Pets in Every Hostel' accreditation scheme in the UK (StreetVet, 2022).

As veterinary nurses, we can utilize our skillset, together with empathy and awareness of all factors that can encompass the lives of our patients, recognizing the value of supporting owners within their home environments, in particular with the delivery of medical care plans prescribed by their veterinary surgeons.

As our patron of animals St Francis of Assisi said, we have been called to heal wounds, to unite what has fallen apart, and to bring home those who have lost their way. Start by doing what is necessary, then what is possible, and suddenly you are doing the impossible (Sweeney, 2019).

3.9   Questions for Further Discussion

1. How aware do you feel you are of the hidden needs of owners and the effect that these can potentially have on patient welfare and access to veterinary care, observing the Equality Act 2010?
2. How do your veterinary practice care plans take into consideration not just the needs of the patient but also the needs of the owner/caregiver, facilitating concordance?

3. What are your thoughts on the role of a veterinary nurse within the community? What do you perceive to be the opportunities and challenges and how do you feel these could be best facilitated?

3.10   Case Study: Tigger

[CF] would like to share the story of a young couple whose beloved cat, Tigger, an 11-year-old male neutered cat, was diagnosed with diabetes mellitus (DM). Tigger was referred to [CF], in her role as a registered veterinary nurse working in the community, under the direction of the veterinary surgeon treating him, to work with his owners to manage this lifelong condition. The aim of [CF]'s role, when working within the community, is to work with animals and their owners in their homes; and for Tigger's owners, it was to give support in the initial stabilization of the DM, with the desire to achieve stabilization to improve both Tigger's and his owners' quality of life. [CF] has personal knowledge of a close family member who has lived with diabetes for 55 years and is acutely aware of their wellbeing challenges through the year, of neuropathy and how it affects their legs and feet, of heart problems linked to the disease, and how, if they get a wound, it is harder to heal with DM, and of the days when their energy is low. This has helped [CF] to relate to the owners of Tigger and the challenges that Tigger might be faced with through his diabetic journey (Mayo Clinic, 2022).

3.10.1   The owners' perspective

We were informed that the condition could be managed with twice-daily insulin injections and our vet demonstrated how to administer these. We were shocked, realizing that this level of care was not going to be easy, but our vet reassured us that there was some support available and referred us to a veterinary nurse working in the community ([CF]), for this.

Tigger was very cooperative with the vet in the clinical setting but once home we realized that the 'one time' demonstration was not sufficient for us to have the confidence to administer the insulin injections competently. Tigger would hear the fridge door opening and insulin-administering device coming out and make a dash for it. He would struggle and, on a few occasions, we ended up missing him completely with the pen. With work being busy, our stress levels at home soared and of course he picked up on this and became more stressed and difficult to handle. It was a vicious circle. We also had a holiday booked and suddenly realized we could no longer just ask neighbours to pop in and help with his care.

[CF] came to our house and spent time showing us how to calm Tigger (and ourselves) and helped us adjust, so that what was stressful became routine. She helped build our confidence by checking how we were doing the injections and

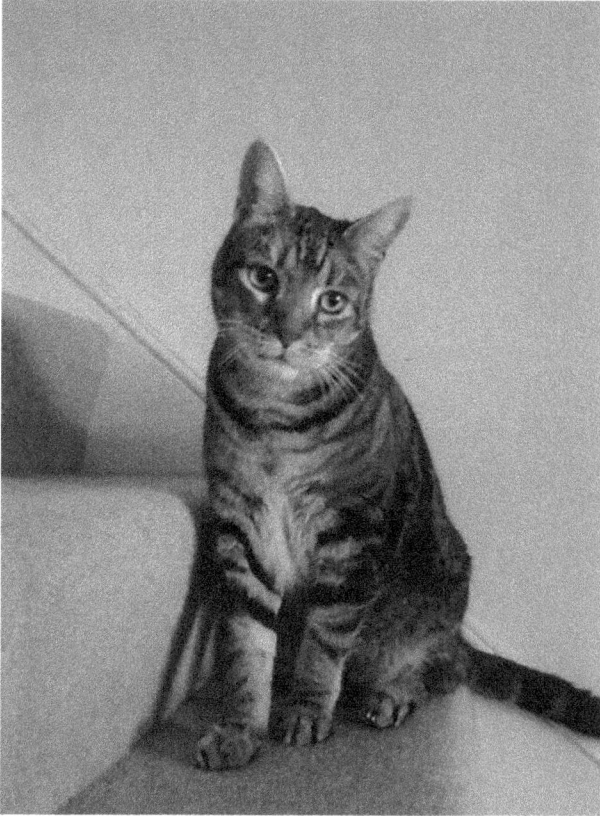

Fig. 3.1. Image of Tigger (used with permission of the owners).

was on hand (when she could be) when we were going away. The quick demonstration in the veterinary clinic, whilst an informative demonstration, was not close to being enough and the visits to our home, as recommended by our vet, made a huge difference.

[CF] continued to help with Tigger's care as his needs became more complex over the following couple of years, but always under the guidance and supervision of our vet. We would have given up on Tigger without her support and we need, without question, more veterinary nurses like her to bridge the gap between vets and the community.

References

Applebaum, J.W., Tomlinson, C.A., Matijczak, A., McDonald, S.E. and Zsembik, B.A. (2020) The concerns, difficulties, and stressors of caring for pets during COVID-19: results from a large survey of U.S. pet owners. *Animals* 10(10), 1882. doi: org/10.3390/ani10101882

Bekoff, M. (2000) Animal emotions: exploring passionate natures: current interdisciplinary research provides compelling evidence that many animals experience such emotions as joy, fear, love, despair, and grief—we are not alone. *BioScience* 50(10), 861–870. doi: 10.1641/0006-3568(2000)050[0861:AEEPN]2.0.CO;2

Blue Cross (2022) *Pet bereavement and pet loss*. Available at: https://www.bluecross. org.uk/pet-bereavement-and-pet-loss (accessed June 2022).

Bowen, J., Bulbena, A. and Fatjó, J. (2021) The value of companion dogs as a source of social support for their owners: findings from a pre-pandemic representative sample and a convenience sample. Obtained during the COVID-19 lockdown in Spain. *Frontiers in Psychiatry* 12, 622060. doi: 10.3389/fpsyt.2021.622060

Brack, G., Franklin, P. and Caldwell, J. (2013) The nurse's role in promoting concordance. In: *Medicines Management for Nursing Practice. Pharmacology, Patient Safety, and Procedure*. Oxford University Press, Oxford, pp. 133–143.

Cocker, F. and Joss, N. (2016) Compassion fatigue among healthcare, emergency and community service workers: a systematic review. *International Journal of Environmental Research and Public Health* 13(6), 618. Available at: https:// pubmed.ncbi.nlm.nih.gov/27338436/ (accessed December 2022).

Dementia Friends (2022) *Champion experience: Carla's story*. Available at: https:// www.dementiafriends.org.uk/WEBNewsStory?storyId=a0B0J00000u3dSR UAY&fbclid=IwAR36u0XtC4RHRFEscapOxSgax4UomZ5jfw2nuvoDSuTx-rzBkKs6gCKhYgA#.Yb81nr3P02y (accessed April 2022).

Endenburg, N. and van Lith, H. (2011) The influence of animals on the development of children. *The Veterinary Journal* 190(2), 208–214.

Equality and Human Rights Commission (2020) Disability discrimination. Available at: https://equalityhumanrights.com/en/advice-and-guidance/disaility-discrimination (accessed August 2022).

ESA (2022) *Emotional Support Animals UK registry*. Available at: https://www. esaorguk.com/ (accessed August 2022)

Gácsi, M., Maros, K., Sernkvist, S., Faragó, T. and Miklósi, Á. (2013) Human analogue safe haven effect of the owner: behavioural and heart rate response to stressful social stimuli in dogs. *PLoS ONE* 8(3), e58475. doi: 10.1371/journal. pone.0058475

Gates, M.C., Walker, J., Zito, S. and Dale, A. (2019) Cross-sectional survey of pet ownership, veterinary service utilisation, and pet-related expenditures in New Zealand. *New Zealand Veterinary Journal* 67(6), 306–314. doi: 10.1080/00480169.2019.1645626

Gee, N.R. and Mueller, M.K. (2019) A systematic review of research on pet ownership and animal interactions among older adults. *Anthrozoös* 32(2), 183–207. doi: 10.1080/08927936.2019.1569903

Glenk, L.M. (2017) Current perspectives on therapy dog welfare in animal-assisted interventions. *Animals* 7(2), 7. doi: 10.3390/ani7020007

Grant, R.A., Montrose, V.T. and Wills, A.P. (2017) ExNOTic: should we be keeping exotic pets? *Animals* 7(6), 47. doi: 10.3390/ani7060047

HABRI (2022a) *Mental health*. Human Animal Bond Research Institute. Available at: https://habri.org/research/mental-health (accessed August 2022).

HABRI (2022b) *Child health and development: autism spectrum disorder*. Human Animal Bond Research Institute Available at: https://habri.org/research/child-health/autism/ (accessed December 2022)

HABRI (2022c) *Mental health: social isolation and loneliness.* Human Animal Bond Research Institute Available at: https://habri.org/research/mental-health/ (accessed December 2022)

HABRI (2022d) *Pet-inclusive housing initiative.* Human Animal Bond Research Institute Available at: https://habri.org/pet-inclusive-housing-initiative (accessed December 2022).

HABRI (2022e) *How does reading to rabbits affect the reading skills of third grade students?* Human Animal Bond Research Institute. Available at: https://habri.org/grants/projects/listening-ears (accessed August 2022)

HOPE Animal-Assisted Crisis Response (2022) *Frequently asked questions.* Available at: https://www.hopeaacr.org/about-hope/frequently-asked-questions (accessed April 2022)

Kennel Club (2020) *The Covid-19 puppy boom – one in four admit impulse buying a pandemic puppy.* Available at: https://www.thekennelclub.org.uk/media-centre/2020/august/the-covid-19-puppy-boom-one-in-four-admit-impulse-buying-a-pandemic-puppy/ (accessed June, 2022)

Kerman, N., Gran-Ruaz, S. and Lem, M. (2019) Pet ownership and homelessness: a scoping review. *Journal of Social Distress and Homelessness* 28(2), 106–114. doi: 10.1080/10530789.2019.1650325

Learning Disability Today (2022) *The benefits of therapeutic horse riding for autistic children.* Available at: https://www.learningdisabilitytoday.co.uk/the-benefits-of-therapeutic-horse-riding-for-autistic-children (accessed April 2022)

Levine, G.N., Allen, K., Braun, L.T., Christian, H.E., Friedmann, E. *et al.* (2013) Pet ownership and cardiovascular risk: a scientific statement from the American Heart Association. *Circulation* 127(23), 2353–2363.

Liu, Z., Heffernan, C. and Tan, J.(2020) Caregiver burden: a concept analysis. *International Journal of Nurse Science* 7(4), 438–445.

Mayo Clinic (2022) *Type-2 diabetes.* Available at: https://www.mayoclinic.org/diseases-conditions/type-2-diabetes/symptoms-causes/syc-20351193 (accessed April 2022)

McNicholas, J., Gilbey, A., Rennie, A., Ahmedzai, S., Dono, J.-A. and Ormerod, E. (2005) Pet ownership and human health: a brief review of evidence and issues. *BMJ* 331, 1252–1254. doi: 10.1136/bmj.331.7527.1252

McNicholas, J. and Collis, G.M. (2000) Dogs as catalysts for social interaction: robustness of the effect. *British Journal of Psychology* 91, 61–70. doi: 10.1348/000712600161673

Melson, G. (2002) Psychology and the study of human–animal relationship. *Society and Animals* 10(4), 347–352.

Noah, D. and Ostrowski, S. (2018) *Zooeyia.* MSD Veterinary Manual. Available at: https://msdvetmanual.com/en-au/zooeyia (accessed August 2020)

Papworth Trust (2018) *Facts and Figures 2018. Disability in the United Kingdom.* Available at: www.papworthtrust.org.uk (accessed August 2022)

PDSA (2022) *Diabetes in dogs.* People's Dispensary for Sick Animals. Available at: https://www.pdsa.org.uk/pet-help-and-advice/pet-health-hub/conditions/diabetes-in-dogs (accessed April 2022)

Pet Partners (2019) *Animal-assisted crisis response.* Pet Partners, Bellevue, Washington. Available at: https://petpartners.org/act/aacr/ (accessed August 2022)

PFMA (2021) *PFMA releases latest pet population data.* Pet Food Manufacturers Association. Available at: https://www.pfma.org.uk/news/pfma-releases-latest-pet-population-data#_edn1 (accessed August 2022)

Price, E.O. (1984) Behavioral aspects of animal domestication. *The Quarterly Review of Biology* 59(1), 1–32.

RCN (2019) *Professional development*. Royal College of Nursing. Available at: https://www.rcn.org.uk/professional-development/publications/pub-007925 (accessed April 2022).

SCAS (2020) *Creating compassionate workplaces: pet bereavement – a guide for employers*. Society for Companion Animal Studies. Available at: http://www.scas.org.uk/wp-content/uploads/2020/01/Creating-Compassionate-Workplaces-January-2020.pdf (accessed June, 2022)

Scoresby, K.J., Strand, E.B., Ng, Z., Brown, K.C., Stilz, C.R. *et al.* (2021) Pet ownership and quality of life: a systematic review of the literature. *Veterinary Science* 8, 332. doi: 10.3390/vetsci8120332

Shubert, J. (2012) Therapy dogs and stress management assistance during disasters. *US Army Medical Department Journal* (April–June), 74+ (1680L)

Staats, S., Wallace, H. and Anderson, T. (2008) Reasons for companion animal guardianship (pet ownership) from two populations. *Society & Animals* 16(3), 279–291. doi: https://doi.org/10.1163/156853008X323411

Stamps, J.A. and Groothuis, T.G.G. (2010) The development of animal personality: relevance, concepts and perspectives. *Biological Reviews* 85, 301–325 doi: 10.1111/j.1469-185X.2009.00103.x

StreetVet (2022) *StreetVet accredited hostel scheme*. Available at: https://www.streetvet.co.uk/streetvet-accredited-hostel-scheme (accessed June 2022)

Sweeney, J. (2019) *Saint Francis of Assisi: His Life, Teachings and Practice*. The Essential Wisdom Library, New York.

Teoh, S.L., Letchumanan, V. and Lee, L.H. (2021) Can Mindfulness help to alleviate loneliness? A systematic review and meta-analysis. *Frontiers in Psychology* 25 (12), 633319. doi: 10.3389/fpsyg.2021.633319

Uccheddu, S., Ronconi, L., Albertini, M., Coren, S., Da Graça Pereira, G. *et al.* (2022) Domestic dogs (*Canis familiaris*) grieve over the loss of a conspecific. *Scientific Reports* 12, 1920. doi: 10.1038/s41598-022-05669-y

Wilson, V., Guenther, A., Øverli, Ø., Seltmann, M.W. and Altschul, D. (2019) Future directions for personality research: contributing new insights to the understanding of animal behavior. *Animals* 9(5), 240. doi: 10.3390/ani9050240

Wood, L., Giles- Corti, B., Bulsara, M. and Bosch, D. (2007) More than a furry companion: the ripple effect of companion animals on neighbourhood interactions and sense of community. *Society and Animals* 15 (1), 43–56.

Zeder, M.A. (2012) The domestication of animals. *Journal of Anthropological Research* 68(2), 161–190.

Other Useful Websites

Cinnamon Trust
National charity for the elderly, the terminally ill and their pets
https://cinnamon.org.uk (accessed June 2022)

Dogs for Good
UK-based charity, training dogs to help adults and children with physical disabilities and learning disabilies, children with autism and adults with dementia (formerly known as Dogs for the Disabled)
https://www.dogsforgood.org (accessed May 2022)

Ehlers-Danos Organisation UK
Charity based in Borehamwood, UK, to support those with Ehlers-Danos sydromes
https://www.ehlers-danlos.org (accessed April 2022)

International Cat Care
Charity based in Tisbury, UK, seeking to improve health and welfare of domestic cats worldwide
https://icatcare.org/advice/diabetes-mellitus/ (accessed April 2022)

Say Aphasia
Charity based in Brighton, UK, offering help and support based on first-hand experience, also aiming to raise awareness and understanding of aphasia
https://www.sayaphasia.org (accessed August 2022)

Non-Communicable Diseases and Other Shared Health Risks[1]

4

Kirsty Cavill[1]*, Nicola Lakeman[2], Robyn Lowe[3], Hayley Burdge[4] and Paula Boyden[5]

[1]*Paws Canine Myotherapy Care, The Vet Connection, UK;* [2]*IVC Evidensia, Bristol, UK;* [3]*Vets 4 Pets, Wigan, UK;* [4]*Langford Vets, Bristol, UK;* [5]*The Links Group, UK*

Key Points

- An introduction to non-communicable diseases
- Examples of non-communicable diseases and the comparative factors between humans and animals
- Examples of other shared health risks

4.1   Introduction

Non-communicable diseases (NCDs), also known as chronic diseases, are diseases that cannot be directly transmitted between people or between animals. According to the World Health Organization (WHO, 2021), NCDs kill 41 million people each year, equivalent to 71% of all deaths globally. Each year, more than 15 million people die from an NCD between the ages of 30 and 69 years; 85% of these 'premature' deaths occur in low- and middle-income countries. Cardiovascular disease alone accounts for 17.9 million deaths annually. NCDs disproportionately affect people in low and low-middle income countries, where more than three-quarters of global NCD deaths occur (WHO, 2021).

In this chapter, we explore the associated and relevant interrelationships within the triad of One Health of a range of NCDs, alongside considering the relevance of non-accidental injury (NAI). NAI is the intentional causing of harm or injury to an animal or person.

It is beyond the scope of this chapter to cover all NCDs, but examples will include osteoarthritis, cardiovascular disease, obesity, passive smoking

---

* Email: pawsmyotherapycare@gmail.com

© CAB International 2023. *One Health for Veterinary Nurses and Technicians*
(eds R. Jones and A. Jeffery)
DOI: 10.1079/9781789249477.0004

and non-accidental injury – examining the links between animal cruelty, child abuse and domestic violence.

It is recognized that humans and companion animals have numerous disease processes in common, including cancer, cardiac, obesity, respiratory and endocrine disease (Natterson-Horowitz *et al.*, 2022). A coordinated collaboration in health research affords the potential to advance the understanding of mutually relevant diseases through a translational approach to health. Disease and health exist within complex molecular, biological, ecological and economic systems. Understanding these dynamic relationships, dependencies and interactions can aid us in recognizing, identifying, treating and preventing these disease processes. Through a collaborative One Health approach, understanding of non-communicable diseases can be advanced.

4.2   Osteoarthritis

Osteoarthritis (OA) is a global disease associated with diverse phenotypes, with variable clinical presentations, rates of progression and responses to therapeutic interventions. It is a common, incurable, progressive and multifactorial disease process of synovial joints, affecting the appendicular and axial skeletal systems, resulting in the breakdown and eventual loss of cartilage in one or more joints. OA is caused by an interplay of risk factors. It is not a single disease but the result of a combination of genetic, physiological, environmental and behavioural factors. It is extremely prevalent in society and is a major cause of disability, affecting millions of humans and companion animals worldwide, resulting in them living with chronic pain and associated disability. OA impairs functionality of the patient and in humans places a burden on individuals and on health and social care systems.

The prevalence of OA in humans is increasing in part due to population ageing and increases in related factors such as obesity (Safiri *et al.*, 2020). The number of people aged over 65 with a musculoskeletal condition in England and Wales is predicted to increase by over 50% by 2030 (The British Geriatric Society, 2015).

There is a developing awareness amongst medical and veterinary professionals and researchers that mutual co-studies of animals and humans could prove beneficial in the development of treatment options, under the One Health umbrella.

The aetiology of OA in humans and animals has some identifiable areas of relative comparability across a multitude of associated risk factors. In humans, systemic and local causes for the development of OA are associated with a variety of both modifiable and non-modifiable risk factors, including age, gender, obesity, lack of exercise, genetic predisposition, previous joint trauma and concurrent underlying disease processes, suggesting that joint disease is a multifactorial disorder.

A systematic review of risk factors conducted by Anderson *et al.* (2020) concluded that osteoarthritis is highly prevalent within the dog population, leading to substantial implications for quality of life and welfare. The review identified the main risk factors in canines as genetics, sex, breed and age (non-modifiable risk factors) with neuter status and body weight identified as modifiable risk factors. An increasing body weight was found to have an association with joint disease, most likely due to the increased load on joints (Anderson *et al.*, 2020).

In comparison, Barbour *et al.* (2017) concluded from a study in North America that the prevalence of arthritis was particularly high among humans with co-morbid conditions, such as heart disease, diabetes and obesity. They reported that almost one-third of all adults who are obese also have arthritis and that 49% of adults with arthritis who are also obese have activity limitations.

Understanding the key risk factors for the development of osteoarthritis in humans and companion animals is essential in identifying prevention and control strategies to reduce prevalence in future generations. Humans and companion animals are often observed to experience shared lifestyle factors and environmental influences and they exhibit similarities in disease progression and ageing. Companion animals may therefore be deemed to be effective sentinels, as they share a common environment and lifestyle attributes with their owners.

Osteoarthritis is the most common joint disease diagnosed in veterinary medicine (Anderson *et al.*, 2018), posing a considerable challenge to companion animal welfare. Canine OA is generally considered to bear a close resemblance to human OA with regard to anatomic similarity, disease heterogeneity and progression. Hannah Capon, founder of Canine Arthritis Management (CAM) – a veterinary-led initiative to raise awareness of canine OA – discussed how canine arthritis is the most common cause of chronic pain in dogs, affecting four out of five older dogs. She went on to say that OA is a disabling, non-curable and progressive disease that initially focuses on moving joints, eventually affects the whole dog and is a major cause of euthanasia due to loss of quality of life (CAM, 2021).

A study by Slingerland *et al.* (2011) concluded that the prevalence of OA in cats is strikingly high and increases with age. Similar studies with dogs have also suggested that osteoarthritis is a disease of ageing and that comparable effects have also been identified in humans (Anderson *et al.*, 2018).

It is estimated that 40% of all cats have clinical signs of OA and 90% of cats over the age of 12 years have radiographic evidence of OA (Lascelles *et al.*, 2010). However, OA in cats is reportedly diagnosed far less frequently in practice, compared with dogs. This is thought to be because cats are presented less often in practice, in comparison with dogs (Lascelles *et al.*, 2010).

The primary complication related to OA is chronic pain. The ability to experience pain is universally shared by all mammals, including companion animals. Similarities in neurophysiology observed across mammals suggest that pain experienced by humans and animals is comparable (Williams, 2019). Chronic pain is recognized to be one of the most disabling effects of OA for both animals and humans diagnosed with this condition. It is maladaptive and representative of a malfunction in neurological transmission and serves no physiological purpose. Chronic or persistent pain entails a pathological reorganization of the neural system and can become the primary symptom in people and animals diagnosed with OA, although in the case of pets, clinical signs may not be always recognized by owners in the early stages of the disease process (Belshaw *et al.*, 2020a,b).

The pain states associated with OA are often complex in nature, involving nociceptive and neuropathic mechanisms. Chronic pain is generally defined as a pain that lasts more than 12 weeks (NHS Inform, 2021a). Chronic musculoskeletal pain is further defined as persistent or recurrent pain arising from a disease affecting the bone, joint, muscle, or related soft tissue. Pain impacts directly on quality of life (QOL) and health-related quality of life, which is a multidimensional concept relating to physical, mental, emotional and social functioning. Therefore, the effects of OA on human, pet and owner are far reaching and inherently interlinked.

The World Small Animal Veterinary Association Global Pain Council (WSAVA GPC, available at: https://wsava.org/committees/global-pain-council, accessed December 2021) recognizes the need to address and eliminate the gap between pain incidence and pain treatment. WSAVA's vision discusses the development of an empowered, motivated and globally unified veterinary profession, which can effectively recognize and minimized pain prevalence and its impact on animals (Matthews *et al.*, 2014).

Breakthrough pain is defined by the WSAVA as an '*abrupt, short-lived, and intense pain that "breaks through" the analgesia that controls pain*'. Therefore, regular assessments and a proactive treatment approach are essential when managing the pain associated with OA. Due to its unpredictable nature and causative factors, pain is broader than just a pharmaceutical solution.

The identification of pain in a companion animal may not always be straightforward or immediately transparent. Pain is often expressed visually rather than vocally in animals; therefore, subtle behavioural or mobility-related changes can be indicative of changing pain states. Lascelles *et al.* (2007) described the use of client-specific outcome measures and activity monitoring to measure the effectiveness of pain relief in cats with OA.

The most common locations of OA in dogs include the stifle, hip, shoulder and elbow, which are common with their homologous equivalent in humans. It can also be noted that the average lifespan of a large-breed dog is 12 years, which equates to a proportionately longer time spent in old age, compared with that of a typical human lifestyle (Fig. 4.1).

As companion animals, notably dogs, share both lifestyle attributes and environments with humans, there are commonalities in the modalities of therapy employed in the treatment of OA across both the human and veterinary care systems. These include pharmaceutical, surgical and non-medical

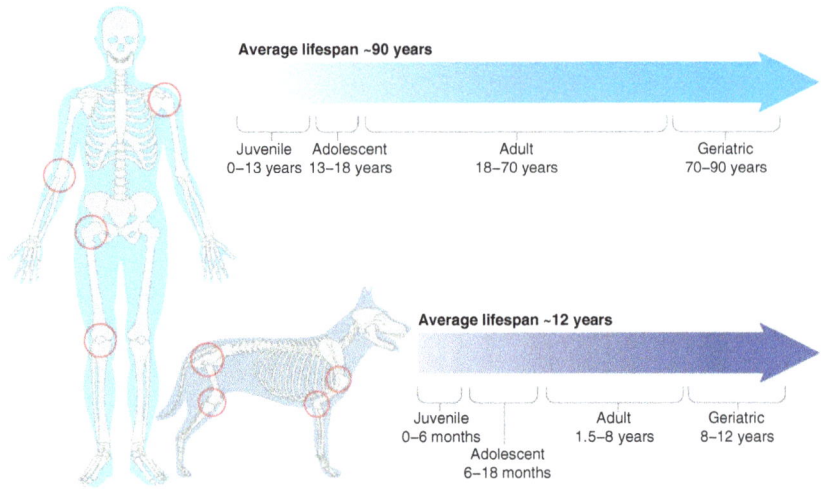

Fig. 4.1. Spontaneous dog osteoarthritis — a One Medicine vision. (With permission of Meeson *et al.*, 2019.)

conservative management options, including physical rehabilitative therapies. These modalities have been shown as effective interventions and there is a collective synergism when used together in a comprehensive and interdisciplinary care model.

Common modalities of treatment options for humans and companion animals diagnosed with OA include therapeutic input (physiotherapy, myotherapy, hydrotherapy, laser therapy) and the use of pharmaceutical medication, alongside exercise, nutrition, weight and lifestyle management plans or surgical intervention.

Regardless of cause, OA has significant physical, social and psychological impacts on patients, both human and animal. Knowledge within the model of OA care is constantly changing and advancing, with the development of new pharmaceuticals and medical and non-medical techniques. Through a better understanding of the disease process, treatment options are developing all the time. The goal of any conservative treatment plan should be to reduce pain, improve quality of life and slow down progression of the disease process.

An additional complication of OA in companion animals is the resulting effect on the caregiver. There is growing awareness that caring for a chronically ill pet may have a detrimental impact on the owner's quality of life through the concept of caregiver burden (see Chapter 3: The Human–Animal Bond). A recent study concluded that caring for an osteoarthritic dog can have multi-faceted, negative impacts on owners which may be sustained over many years, particularly if the dog is young at diagnosis (Belshaw *et al.*, 2020a,b).

Registered Veterinary Nurses (RVNs) must remain mindful of the impact associated with QOL for both patient and owner and also protect themselves from the effects of burden transfer, which can affect the client–vet/nurse bond, medication compliance, patient outcome, quality of life and longevity.

In terms of global burden and prevalence, OA is a major public and animal health challenge and whilst there is a wide variation in prevalence in humans globally, the burden is increasing in most countries. A systematic analysis of the Global Burden of Disease study 2017 concluded that raising policy-maker awareness of risk factors, which include body weight and injury, and the importance and benefits of management of OA, together with providing health services for an increasing number of people living with OA, are recommended for management of the future burden of this condition (Safiri *et al.*, 2020).

Patient-centred care and pursuing the objective of best available practices that employ a multisectoral and transdisciplinary approach are an effective approach in the management of OA and are recognized as modalities which transcend the concept of One Health. By proactively investing in the targeted development of evidence-based and nurse-centric care plans, patients can be effectively monitored and the condition proactively managed.

There is recognition across the veterinary profession that weight management has a role to play in many disease processes. There are two mechanisms by which obesity can exacerbate the clinical signs of OA: (i) a *physical* effect from the forces experienced by an affected joint; and (ii) *biologically* from the active nature of adipose tissue. Adipokines, a mixture of hormones and biochemical molecules produced by adipose tissue, are pro-inflammatory in nature and may therefore trigger a low-grade inflammatory state, potentially contributing to the joint damage.

Weight management and the clinical and physical effects of obesity, including the relationship with diabetes and cardiovascular disease, are embedded in both human and veterinary medicine and are therefore often the focus of a One Health model.

4.3 Obesity

Prevalence rates of obesity in human and animal populations are increasing rapidly. Pets and people share several obesity-related co-morbidities. Obesity is a major risk factor for type 2 diabetes mellitus in people and in cats, but this association is not recognized in dogs (Chandler *et al.*, 2017).

There have been numerous studies looking into the behaviour of pet owners as caregivers to the animal and comparison with childhood obesity. Obesity is a very complex condition; it is not just about what you eat. There are so many overlapping elements of food, exercise, emotions, social economics and learnt feeding behaviours. Notable parallels exist between human and companion animal obesity, and this is not surprising for outbred species sharing the same environment (German, 2015).

People who live with pets harbour a different gastrointestinal microbiota to those who do not own a pet (Arenas-Montes *et al.*, 2021); this shaping of the microbiota might influence the prevalence of cardiovascular disease, metabolic syndrome and obesity in humans. Links have been made to pet ownership influencing obesity rates in humans – the gut biome in humans and in turn dermatological conditions and obesity and even how owning a pet can influence the care people give themselves in terms of their own healthcare (Maranda and Gupta, 2016). The relationship between the risk of cardiovascular disease and owning pets has not been sufficiently studied, although being in contact with pets has been considered a protective factor against cardiovascular disease (Levine *et al.*, 2013; Yeh *et al.*, 2019) and other diseases in children, including allergies and obesity (Azad *et al.*, 2013; Tun *et al.*, 2017). Some evidence suggests that this protection might be due to favourable changes in the intestinal microbiota (Arenas-Montes *et al.*, 2021).

Obesity in pets may be an intriguing model for childhood obesity. The care that owners provide for their pets can mirror that which is provided for children. Owners of obese pets tend to over-humanize them (Kienzle *et al.*, 1998; Kienzle and Bergler, 2006), with pets being viewed as a substitute child (Charles and Davies, 2008). Dogs owned by overweight people are more likely to be overweight than the dogs of owners who are not overweight (Holmes *et al.*, 2007) and, as is the case with parents misperceiving the body shape of their children, misperception of the body shape is also seen in pet owners (Courcier *et al.*, 2011). Owners 'normalize' their animal's body condition, where most owners of overweight dogs underestimate their dog's body condition (Courcier *et al.*, 2011). Understanding parental styles and their impact on childhood obesity can help understand the complexities of owner and pet and how childhood obesity strategies can be utilized in the veterinary industry.

Pet owner risk factors for canine and feline obesity include owner household income and exercise habits (Courcier *et al.*, 2010).

One Health is a term that we regularly hear in veterinary press but what is our role in promoting it? What does this mean for RVNs in veterinary practice, especially in terms of obesity? Our role is not to instigate obesity clinics for our clients, but we do need to be mindful that owner education regarding the prevention and management of obesity can have a positive effect on the pet owner's health and wellbeing. We should not be afraid to discuss these elements. Using human weight-loss digital aids to monitor the pet can be helpful. The use of exercise trackers or food diaries can be very helpful to track the amount of exercise that dogs have undertaken. Some owners will start using these for themselves when they start seeing the advantages. Taking elements from human weight-loss medicine can benefit veterinary medicine. We know from human behavioural studies that motivation and support from others is a vital aspect in the success of weight-loss programmes. Having a structured nutritional plan with meal schedules also benefits, alongside monitoring of exercise levels.

It has been proposed that implementing a One-Health-for-obesity approach could provide several benefits in comparison with 'silo approaches', because sharing of knowledge and experience could strengthen the message, helping to reach a larger audience (Häsler *et al.*, 2014).

Understanding the environmental, genetic and behavioural origins of diseases known to be shared across species can help us improve and expand the tools available for their prevention and management (Rijnberk *et al.*, 2003). A One Health view on the obesity (and co-morbidities) crisis can spur innovative and novel approaches by bringing together engaged groups of people to take meaningful roles in supporting individuals in promoting their health and the health of their pet (Chandler *et al.*, 2017).

4.4 Cardiovascular Disease

4.4.1 Comparative aetiology

Cardiovascular disease (CVD) is the leading cause of death worldwide, accounting for 45% of all deaths (> 4 million) in Europe (Mubanga *et al.*, 2017). In the UK, CVD prevalence in humans has remained constant at around 3% in England and 4% in Scotland, Wales and Northern Ireland. CVD mortality in the UK is declining but the burden on health care comes not only from deaths, but also from the implications of living with the disease, with hospital admissions increasing (Bhatnagar *et al.*, 2016) and from the associated costs.

The aetiology of CVD in animals and humans is relatively incomparable, with humans commonly experiencing coronary heart disease, atherosclerosis and atheroma commonly linked to obesity. Dogs are represented with degenerative valve disease and acquired cardiomyopathies, with cardiomyopathies being most prevalent in cats (Collins, 2016), with specific risk factors making some individuals more predisposed to specific disease processes.

When assessing One Health and cardiovascular health we can draw in multiple factors for humans and companion animals as to the negative and positive influences on CVD with regard to social factors, beliefs, environmental implications and the human–animal bond. As veterinary professionals, taking into consideration human, animal and environmental factors will help provide holistic care, aid in compliance in treatment options that will benefit the patient's health and welfare and allow greater owner satisfaction and engagement.

4.4.2 Brachycephalic pet ownership

Brachycephalic pet ownership has increased over recent years in feline, canine and lagomorph populations (Farnworth *et al.*, 2018; O'Neill *et al.*, 2019). The Royal Veterinary College (RVC, 2021) believes that understanding the motivations and desires of current and prospective brachycephalic owners is key in devising more targeted human behaviour change interventions in the future for the benefit of the animals' health and welfare. The rising popularity and ownership over the past decade of the Pug, French Bulldog and British Bulldog has been central to growing concerns about brachycephalic health issues in dogs. Owners of brachycephalic breeds are noted to be motivated to acquire their pet primarily based on their appearance, with important factors such as breed health or longevity having a lesser influence on their breed choice (Packer *et al.*, 2017). There is strong evidence to support the common claim that brachycephalic breeds are generally less healthy than their non-brachycephalic counterparts (O'Neill, 2020). Brachycephalic syndrome is characterized by the combination of primary and secondary upper respiratory tract abnormalities and may result in significant upper airway obstruction. These changes lead to increased resistance of the air passages, which can cause elevation of pulmonary pressure and clinical manifestations attributable to pulmonary hypertension. The consequence of this secondary respiratory distress is right-sided cardiac remodelling (cor pulmonale) with possible progression to right-sided congestive heart failure (Canola *et al.*, 2018). Education attempts to improve breed health and public perception of brachycephalic health and welfare are ongoing by the profession.

4.4.3 Pet ownership and social prescribing

Dog ownership may be beneficial in reducing cardiovascular risk in their owners by providing social support and motivation for physical activity. A study by Mubanga *et al.* (2017) indicated that dog ownership was associated with a lower risk of incident cardiovascular disease in single-person households and with lower cardiovascular and all-cause mortality in the general population.

Pet ownership in general has also been suggested to be a marker of better socioeconomic status and family stability (Schreiner, 2016). If companion animals reduce the risk of CVD, then looking at local and national improved educational prospects for lower socioeconomic groups, the use of social prescribing in appropriate households and opportunity for considered and sensible pet ownership could be considered. Worryingly, a report by the Social Mobility Commission (2016) found that in areas vital to child development and attainment at school, gaps were widening between high and low socioeconomic status families when it comes to several factors. The risk of CVD and mortality is reduced by alleviating psychosocial stress factors, such as social isolation, depression and loneliness – all reportedly lower in dog owners (Mubanga *et al.*, 2017). Furthermore, it has consistently been shown that dog owners achieve more physical activity and spend more time engaged in outdoor activities (Mubanga *et al.*, 2017).

4.4.4 'Natural is best' belief system

It is common for concepts in human health trends to leak into those of veterinary medicine. In human healthcare, the belief that 'natural' medications are better, healthier and safer than synthetic drugs is a regular occurrence, and researchers have found that these beliefs, or biases, affect the decisions people make about their health (NCCIH, 2022). This can also translate to their decision making in their pets.

One common way this translates is regarding decisions about what diet owners provide for their pets. There are some nutritional inadequacies being noted due to certain 'boutique' diets, grain-free diets, raw diets, nutritionally unbalanced home prepared foods and owners providing vegan diets to obligate carnivore species.

In a study by Adin *et al.* (2019) looking at echocardiographic phenotype of canine dilated cardiomyopathy (DCM), it was found that left ventricle size in diastole and systole is greater and sphericity index is less in common grain-free diets compared with grain-based diets, suggesting that those on the grain-free diets had more severe cardiac remodelling in comparison with the grain-based diet group. In a study by Freid *et al.* (2021), dogs with DCM eating non-traditional diets experienced improvement in cardiac function after diet change. Survival time was significantly longer for dogs with DCM eating non-traditional diets that had their diets changed, compared with dogs eating non-traditional diets that did not have their diets changed. Additional research is needed to examine possible associations between diet and DCM (Freid *et al.*, 2021).

4.4.5 Environmental contaminants

Since around the 1980s, hyperthyroidism in cats has increased from 1 in 200 to around 1 in 10; this epidemic may be linked to exposure to a chemical contained in flame retardants commonly found in furniture (McReynolds, 2019). Cardiovascular abnormalities are relatively common in hyperthyroid cats, although the severity and prevalence have decreased in recent years, presumably because of earlier diagnosis and effective treatment options. While hyperthyroidism most commonly induces a reversible form of hypertrophic cardiomyopathy, a dilative type has also been described and overt congestive cardiac failure can arise from either, albeit uncommonly. A study by Poutasse *et al.* (2019) into hyperthyroidism in cats led researchers to think about hyperthyroidism in humans. Even at the cellular level, the benign tumour associated with feline hyperthyroidism is comparable in cats and humans. Extrapolating from this, hyperthyroid cats could be an indicator for humans, warning of a possible link between flame retardants and human hyperthyroidism. However, the evidence does not allow us to draw conclusions and future studies will possibly shed light on this concept of the environmental impact of fire-retardant chemicals on the thyroid and subsequently cardiac health.

Non-communicable diseases are examples of how the health of humans and companion animals is intrinsically linked. Their shared living environments and lifestyles means that they are also subject to other shared health risks. One such example is passive smoking.

4.5   Passive Smoking

It is well known that smoking has many harmful effects to human health. However, it is not only the smoker who is being put at risk. Inhalation of environmental tobacco smoke or second-hand smoke from the burning end of a cigarette or smoke that is exhaled by the smoker is also harmful. This is known as passive smoking. The NHS states, '*People exposed to second-hand smoke face the same dangers as smokers themselves*' (NHS Inform, 2020).

Second-hand smoke contains more than 7000 chemicals, of which hundreds are toxic and approximately 70 are believed to be carcinogenic (CDC, 2021). Even brief exposure to second-hand smoke can be harmful to health. Adults who breathe in second-hand smoke have an increased risk of heart disease, stroke and lung cancer. It has been documented that people who do not smoke but are exposed to second-hand smoke at home or at work experience a 25–30% increase in their risk of developing heart disease (CDC, 2021). In the USA, second-hand smoke exposure causes more than 7300 deaths from lung cancer among people who do not smoke and more than 8000 deaths from stroke each year can be attributed to second-hand smoke (CDC, 2021).

The UK Government's Scientific Committee on Tobacco and Health (SCOTH) reported in November 2004 that exposure to second-hand smoke was a '*substantial public health hazard*' (ASH, 2015). The 'Smoke Free law' was enforced in July 2007, forbidding smoking in enclosed public spaces, including public transport, work vehicles and company cars.

Most second-hand smoke is invisible and odourless and can linger for up to 5 hours after the cigarette is extinguished (NHS, 2021) and the second-hand smoke in the environment is absorbed into permeable surfaces, such as furniture and upholstery. This is also known as third-hand smoke, and will accumulate in dust and get trapped in carpets and other porous materials (Kramer *et al.*, 2004).

Infants and young children are at a particularly high risk from the effects of second-hand smoke, due to their immature respiratory and immune systems and faster respiratory rates. This makes them more susceptible to the harmful chemicals in second-hand smoke (NHS Inform, 2020). Additionally, babies and children are more likely to encounter nicotine in the form of third-hand smoke from residual nicotine found on contaminated surfaces, subsequently leading to the ingestion of further toxic particles. Children exposed to tobacco smoke have a higher prevalence of respiratory symptoms such as coughing, wheezing and shortness of breath. Bronchitis and pneumonia are more likely to occur compared with children living in a smoke-free household (CDC, 2021). Children with pre-existing asthma will have more severe, frequent asthma attacks in a smoking environment (CDC, 2021).

Second-hand smoke cannot easily be confined; it can travel and migrate throughout its environment. The particles are smaller than dust and drift easily through the house and open doors. Restricting smoking to one room or having the window or door open will not reduce the harm (NHS Inform, 2021b). Equally, second-hand smoke can reach dangerous levels inside vehicles; even with windows open or air conditioning on, harmful particles can remain in the atmosphere long after the visible smoke has disappeared (NHS Inform, 2021b). Therefore, it is now against the law to smoke in a private vehicle if there is a young person present under the age of 18 (NHS Inform, 2021b).

Smoking also has a huge negative affect on our environment and the world in which we live in. Tobacco production contributes to deforestation and carbon dioxide pollution. Data shows that 600 million trees are chopped down every year for tobacco production and that one tree will be destroyed for every 15 packs of cigarettes smoked. It takes 4 miles of paper every hour to wrap and package cigarettes and the US tobacco industry produces a staggering 16 million tonnes of carbon dioxide in one year (Tobacco Free Life, 2016).

Cigarette butts are harmful to the environment and to the animals that encounter them, but 4.5 trillion cigarette butts are disposed of each year (EarthDay, 2020), half of which will end up in landfills, with the other half ending up in soil, lakes, oceans and forests. This puts the animals found in these environments at risk from nicotine poisoning. The most affected are beach-dwellers – large turtles, sea cows and seals. They frequently visit contaminated beaches where they eat, and feed their young with, cigarette butts. Scientists have also found cigarette butts in stomachs of hundreds of other species such as birds, cats, dogs and others (Tobacco Free Life, 2016).

In the UK, there are around 6.9 million adults who smoke cigarettes (ONS, 2020) and approximately 59% of households own a pet (Statista, 2021). Pets living in a smoking household could be as vulnerable as children, due to comparable predispositions and behaviours such as faster respiratory rates, being closer to the ground and in frequent contact with high-touch surfaces. Therefore, they are more likely to inhale more of the toxic second-hand smoke and are equally likely to ingest (by licking and chewing) third-hand smoke particles that have been absorbed into the soft furnishings and toys around the home (Ka *et al.*, 2014). Furthermore, evidence shows that nicotine can be absorbed into an animal's fur, which they will then orally ingest during self-grooming (Bawazeer *et al.*, 2012).

We know that exposure to environmental tobacco smoke increases the risk of cancer in both smokers and non-smoking humans. Research also shows that the prevalence of cancer is increased in animals living in a smoking household. Dolichocephalic breeds of dog that are regularly exposed to tobacco smoke will have an increased risk of developing a nasal tumour (Reif *et al.*, 1998), with the risk of developing a nasal tumour being 2.5-fold greater than in mixed-breed dogs (Hayes *et al.*, 1982). It is understood this is due to the larger surface area in their nasal cavity, allowing smoke and particles to be trapped (Hayes *et al.*, 1982), and due them having a greater filtration within their nasal cavity, allowing particles to get impacted in the mucosa (Reif *et al.*, 1998). Conversely, brachycephalic-nosed breeds are more likely to develop lung cancer, because smoke is not filtered in the nose but goes directly into the lungs (Reif *et al.*, 1998).

Two studies concluded that cats living in a smoking household were more likely to develop malignant lymphoma or oral squamous cell carcinoma

(Bertone *et al.*, 2002). This increased risk was associated with both duration and quantity of environmental tobacco smoke exposure; cats living in households in which a pack or more of cigarettes was smoked per day had a significant threefold increase in risk (Bertone *et al.*, 2002). A second study stated that cats that had ever lived in a household with a smoker had a twofold increased risk of oral squamous cell carcinoma and the risk was even higher in cats that had lived with a smoker for 5 or more years and in those that lived with two or more smokers (Snyder *et al.*, 2004).

Reinero *et al.* (2009) suggested that humans and cats may react in similar ways to similar allergens. In humans, persistent exposure to second-hand smoke will increase the incidence of bronchial asthma and research indicates that this is also true in the cat population (Byers and Dhupa, 2005). Studies have demonstrated an association between passive smoking and atopic dermatitis in children (Kim *et al.*, 2017) and in dogs (Ka *et al.*, 2014).

All pets living in a smoking household will breathe in the same toxic toxins produced by environmental tobacco smoke. Birds are extremely sensitive, due to their small size and well-developed respiratory system. They will also ingest these toxins whilst preening themselves, similarly to cats whilst grooming. Birds have been shown to develop respiratory illness, feather plucking, allergies, sinus, skin, eye and fertility problems, cancers and heart disease from exposure to cigarette smoke. Mice, guinea pigs and other small pets will suffer from respiratory problems, such as emphysema, and vascular disease because of exposure to smoke. Fish can also be affected, as the toxins from the smoke can be easily dissolved into water and even small quantities can be deadly (RSPCA, 2019).

Nicotine found in cigarettes, cigarette butts, e-cigarettes (the device itself, nicotine canisters and refill liquids), nicotine gum and patches poses a risk if ingested. It is therefore imperative that all items and their waste products are kept out of reach of animals to prevent nicotine poisoning.

We have fantastic resources and opportunities to learn and collaborate with our healthcare counterparts to support the One Health concept. A collaboration between the Royal College of Nursing (RCN) and the British Veterinary Nursing Association (BVNA) as part of the VN Futures initiative initiated a One Health approach to support smoking cessation (BVA, 2019).

A smoke-free setting would be ideal for all our animals, humans and the environment. However, this is not always easy to achieve. Therefore, it is imperative that we are equipped with evidence-based knowledge and undergo appropriate training to confront these potentially sensitive conversations. Websites such as the National Centre for Smoking Cessation and Training (NCSCT) (available at: https://www.ncsct.co.uk/, accessed April 2022) are an excellent resource that could be utilized by RVNs to support awareness campaigns and for generating waiting-room literature.

The final section in this chapter will address an aspect of One Health that can have a significant impact on human and animal health. Non-accidental injury is an important area in which all healthcare professionals can play a vital role to improve the welfare of those under their care. It is also one that demonstrates again the interlinks between human and animal health and welfare.

4.6   Non-Accidental Injury (NAI)

4.6.1   An overview of abuse

As a caring profession, it may be difficult to comprehend why someone would deliberately hurt an animal and then seek veterinary attention. Sadly, some people do and this intentional or so-called non-accidental injury (NAI) may be part of a bigger picture, involving the domestic abuse of humans. Whist we cannot definitively say that the person who abuses their partner will abuse the family pet (or vice versa), if there is evidence of abuse it should raise suspicion of the possibility of wider abuse. '*When animals are abused, people are at risk. When people are abused, animals are at risk*' (Arkow, 1994).

With regard to domestic abuse and pets, perpetrators of domestic abuse will utilize the strong bond between an owner and their pet to exert power and control over their victim, via the threat of or actual harm to the pet. Some perpetrators will even buy a pet for their victim, allow a bond to develop, and then subsequently exert coercive control. Understandably, some victims delay fleeing a violent situation if they cannot take their pet with them, for fear of the repercussions on the pet. Hence pet fostering services for the pets of people fleeing domestic abuse are vital for the safety of those affected.

When referring to the term abuse, one might automatically think of physical abuse, or NAI – the terms are synonymous. However, it is important to recognize that there are other forms of abuse. For us to consider abuse in animals, we must not only be able to recognize the abuse, but also use the correct and appropriate terminology. In the case of companion animals, the tried and tested child abuse terminology is used to avoid confusion both within and between professions. The recognized categories of abuse are:

- Physical
- Sexual
- Emotional
- Neglect

Domestic abuse can also include, but is not limited to, coercive control, financial or economic abuse, harassment, stalking and online or digital abuse (Women's Aid, 2021).

It should be no surprise that there are similarities between the abuse of humans and the abuse of animals regarding the circumstances of the violence, the actions involved and the excuses offered. This is due to one common denominator: the human perpetrator. However, these similarities may be difficult for some to understand.

Thanks to the work of Munro and Thrusfield (2001a–d) we now have diagnostic indicators for NAI in a pet. The indicators are the same for NAI in a child (Table 4.1). Certain patterns of injury may also be seen, for example cigarette burns. If a patient is admitted for investigation, be alert for old, unexplained injuries such as rib fractures.

Table 4.1. Diagnostic indicators for non-accidental injuries in a pet.

Indicator	Comments
History inconsistent with the injury	Generally, the injury is too severe for the history given
Discrepant history	The same person giving a different story to different members of the veterinary team, or different members of the family giving different stories to the veterinary team
Repetitive injuries	Should give a strong index of suspicion. Also consider clients who have had numerous pets, especially if the pets have not been seen for some time and it is not known what has happened to them
Behaviour of owner (parent) and/or pet (child)	This is in combination with one or more of the above three factors

4.6.2 The role of the veterinary nurse

Arkow (1994) highlighted that there was growing evidence of a link between violence to people and violence to animals and that veterinarians were important because they see the results of the violence in their animal patients. Experience over the years has highlighted the importance of the veterinary nurse (VN) who might be central in such cases.

- Some clients will speak much more openly to VNs and support staff than they will to a veterinary surgeon; they can therefore be a key source of information.
- Whilst we speak of clients 'vet shopping' between practices, they might also vet shop *within* a practice. The VN may well be the constant if the same patient is hospitalized on several occasions, or if more than one animal from the same household is hospitalized at different times.

It is important that suspected cases of NAI are discussed with those who have encountered the client within the practice team. Cases may be complex and challenging and as much information as possible should be gathered to decide how to proceed.

Whilst our primary responsibility is to our animal patients, as a trusted profession, members of the veterinary team may well be in the position of receiving information about abuse of a human, referred to as disclosure, and we need to know what to do. Showing empathy and compassion towards a suspected human victim of abuse might be the first time anyone has acted in this way and could be a turning point for them to seek help.

Whether faced with a patient with a suspected NAI, or a human victim of abuse, it is important that no one steps outside their area of expertise but that, where possible, concerns are reported accordingly.

4.6.3   Case management

All practices should have their own protocol on how to deal with a suspected case of abuse, whether the victim is an animal or a human. The Links Group guidance document (available at https://thelinksgroup.org.uk/veterinary-team-guidance, accessed August 2022) can be used as a starting point for practices to develop their own protocol.

As part of this it is recommended that each practice has a 'links adviser', the go-to individual within the practice who can collate available information regarding a particular case. The links adviser might fall under a broader safe-guarding responsibility or may be considered a separate role. The nominated individual does not have to be a veterinary surgeon and could be another senior member of staff. In addition to collating information, the links adviser would have knowledge of local agencies that can be accessed, such as domestic abuse services and pet fostering services.

4.6.4   Reporting

The RCVS Code of Professional Conduct supporting guidance (RCVS, 2021) recognizes the part that VNs might play in cases of NAI. The supporting guidance is the same for both vets and VNs regarding client confidentiality, as follows:

> *'14.6 In circumstances where the client has not given permission for disclosure and the veterinary surgeon or veterinary nurse considers that animal welfare or the public interest is compromised, client confidentiality may be breached, and appropriate information reported to the relevant authorities.'*

Possible examples are then listed, including the following:

- An animal shows signs of abuse.
- Child or domestic abuse is suspected.

The guidance goes on to say:

> *'14.9 Veterinary nurses employed by a veterinary surgeon or practice should discuss the issues with a senior veterinary surgeon in the practice before breaching client confidentiality.'*

Reporting suspected cases of NAI of animals is usually to the local SPCA (RSPCA in England and Wales, SSPCA in Scotland) or Animal Welfare Officer (Northern Ireland). Such reports are confidential. Attending veterinary surgeons might be asked to give a statement on an animal they have treated. The source of a report is confidential and will not be disclosed.

For human victims of domestic abuse, one of the most dangerous times for them is around the point of leaving a violent situation. Therefore, whilst a victim might be encouraged to seek help, reports should only be made if they are in immediate danger (in which case call 999). The practice can offer support by having knowledge of local domestic abuse services to be able to signpost.

It is also possible to report concerns via the independent charity Crimestoppers (available at: https://crimestoppers-uk.org, accessed August 2022); this again is confidential, with Crimestoppers not wishing to know the caller's name.

Whilst domestic abuse is a gendered crime (more than one in four women will experience domestic abuse in their lifetime), men can also be victims. It is also important to consider the impact on children; an estimated 62% of children in violent homes are directly harmed (CAADA, 2014). In light of these figures, bear in mind that some members of the practice team might also be impacted by domestic abuse; consideration should be given to what support might be put in place for colleagues.

4.6.5 Summary

Abuse is a complex subject; cases are not straightforward and can be emotionally challenging.

VNs play an integral role in cases and may be the recipients of disclosure about abuse.

Veterinary professionals are not mandated to report suspected abuse of animals or humans, but there are ethical and moral aspects to consider.

4.7 Chapter Summary

There are often inherent links between concurrent disease processes. Therefore, from the perspective of the RVN, it is important to remain mindful of the benefits that can be achieved for patients through the utilization of evidence-based nursing, collaboration and from the identification of clear objectives and procedures to enable the development of effective care plans. The initiation of a proactive approach, in the early stages of the disease process, and recognizing the need to employ a multidisciplinary 'toolbox' of treatment options is beneficial in the long-term management of these patients. RVNs are therefore instrumental in the provision of nurse-led clinics, ensuring owner compliance, removing barriers to clinic attendance, pro-active patient monitoring and community-based care for patients diagnosed with non-communicable diseases, other shared health risk or those at risk from non-accidental injury.

4.8 Questions for Further Discussion

1. Aside from the examples given in this chapter, what other non-communicable disease or health risks do humans and animal share?

2. Animals can act as sentinels for human health risks and vice versa. What is your understanding of this term and can you think of any examples?

3. The similarities in disease progression between companion animals and humans means that they are now recognized as more clinically relevant research models for human diseases than rodents in the field of comparative medicine. What do you understand about comparative medicine and the research under this umbrella?

4.9 Case Study: StreetVet and Shyia the Staffordshire Bull Terrier (SBT)

K. Cavill, BSc (Hons) RVN Canine Myotherapist
StreetVet – Registered Veterinary Charity 1181527

StreetVet (SV) started in 2016, inspired by the incredible bond between a homeless man and his dog. It operates in 17 locations across the UK, with vets and nurses working voluntarily with outreach organizations in multiple communities. It was born out of respect and a will of veterinary professionals to help make a difference to the lives of those living with and experiencing homelessness. Through the utilization of interprofessional collaboration, SV offers the highest level of care by implementing multidisciplinary treatment plans to effectively manage cases.

Current statistics suggest that around 320,000 people are experiencing homelessness in the UK and a significant number of them are homeless with a pet. Rough sleeping is probably the most visible and dangerous form of homelessness.

The bond between human and animal is explicit and beautiful, but the bond between people experiencing homelessness and their dogs is even more profound, such that their pets' wellbeing is a life-shaping priority.

4.9.1 Hostel Accreditation Scheme

SV works closely with hostels around the UK to provide support in ten key areas, enabling the hostels to implement positive pet policies (Fig. 4.2).

Research has shown that fewer than 7% of homeless pet owners would give up their dog in exchange for housing, yet only 10% of all UK hostel projects currently accept pets (Dogs Trust, 2022). SV teams liaise closely with hostels to ensure that accommodation is accessible to both the owner and their pet. The scheme also gives support and training to hostel staff, ensuring that no resident should ever have to leave their pet to access a place of safety.

4.9.2 Shyia, SBT Female. DOB 2008

May 2018

Shyia was first presented to the SV team on an evening outreach session in 2018. Her owner was a young man, experiencing homelessness following the loss of a parent and subsequent family break-up. Shyia had been in her owner's possession

Continued

Case study Continued.

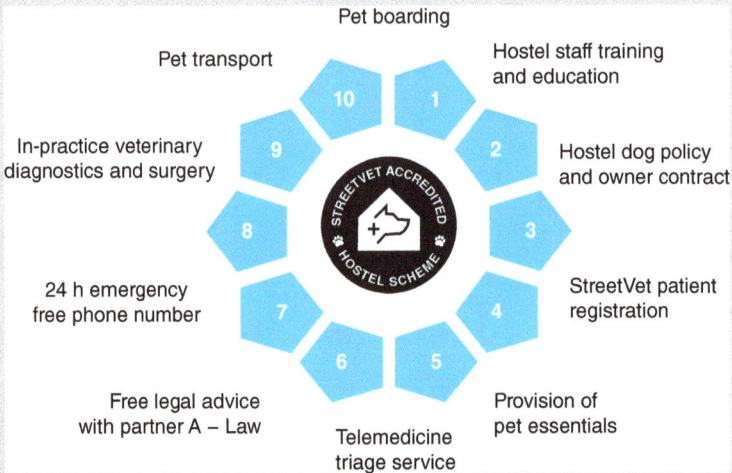

Pet boarding

Pet transport

Hostel staff training
and education

In-practice veterinary
diagnostics and surgery

Hostel dog policy
and owner contract

StreetVet patient
registration

24 h emergency
free phone number

Free legal advice
with partner A – Law

Provision of
pet essentials

Telemedicine
triage service

STREETVET ACCREDITED
HOSTEL SCHEME

10 1 9 2 8 3 7 4 6 5

Fig. 4.2. StreetVet Accredited Hostel Scheme (courtesy of StreetVet).

for 3 years and the mutual bond was apparent to see. Shyia was a lively and happy girl, well socialized and confident.

On initial assessment, the owner reported that Shyia was occasionally a little stiff after rest, but otherwise well. Shyia was started on a course of vaccinations. No lameness was observed and her gait appeared normal. Microchip details were checked and Shyia was given an SV ID tag.

Shyia was seen regularly when her owner attended the soup kitchen.

September 2018
Shyia presented as slightly subdued and her owner reported that she was stiff after walks. On examination, Shyia was exhibiting a wide hind limb stance but otherwise nothing abnormal was detected. The agreed plan was for rest, gentle mobilization and a gradual introduction back to short periods of controlled exercise.

Re-assessment after 1 week: Shyia's owner reported that she was back to normal and no longer showing any signs of stiffness. Nothing abnormal was detected on examination.

December 2018
Shyia's owner had noticed a small lump on her abdomen. Fine-needle aspiration was performed and sent for analysis.

January 2019
Preoperative blood samples were taken and a surgical procedure for ovariohysterectomy and removal of mammary lumps was performed.

May 2019
Shyia was presented with hind limb stiffness. She was assessed and prescribed nutraceuticals and an appropriate analgesia, and a blood sampling protocol was

Continued

Case study Continued.

started to establish baseline parameters. Shyia was referred for myotherapy – a form of physical rehabilitation therapy and clinical massage.

4.9.3 Rehabilitation assessment

Shyia presented with an exaggerated hind limb stance and myofascial trigger points were palpable in the thoracolumbar region, with some restricted range of motion in her stifle joints. Shyia was usually an active dog, regularly walking long distances.

Shyia received regular sessions of myotherapy, to which she responded positively. Her owner was shown some basic massage techniques to use between sessions. Shyia was initially reviewed every 2 weeks and her medication reassessed by the veterinary team regularly. Her mobility improved, she exhibited less muscular stiffness and the trigger points were no longer palpable.

Exercise, lifestyle and weight management plans were discussed. Shyia was fitted with a harness and given an orthopaedic bed and a warm coat. Her owner was dedicated in ensuring he carried out her massage regularly. Treatment plan compliance was never an issue.

4.9.4 Ongoing care

Shyia was presented regularly at outreach sessions for physical therapy and health checks. Due to their unwavering bond, her owner was exceptionally perceptive and would contact SV as soon he noticed any changes.

As Shyia turned 13, there was a noticeable decline in her mobility and changes in her kidney function were identified. Blood and urine parameters were assessed regularly, and her medications reviewed at each outreach by the vet/nurse team. Shyia was started on a renal diet, her medication regime altered accordingly, and her myotherapy sessions continued.

Sadly, in November 2021, Shyia was euthanized due to a concurrent disease process. She passed away peacefully with the SV team members and her owner present. The dedication from her owner was unwavering from his first point of contact with StreetVet, enabling the successful implementation of a multimodal, interprofessional treatment approach to support Shyia's mobility through her senior years. Shyia and her owner had over 40 points of contact with the team following registration in 2018. The SV team continue to support her owner as he adjusts to life without his beloved companion.

Note

[1] Different sections in this chapter were written by different authors as follows: Introduction and Osteoarthritis by Kirsty Cavill; Obesity by Nicola Lakeman; Cardiovascular Disease by Robyn Lowe; Passive Smoking by Hayley Burdge; and Non-Accidental Injury by Paula Boyden.

References

Adin, D., DeFrancesco, T.C., Keene, B., Tou, S., Meurs, K. *et al.* (2019) Echocardiographic phenotype of canine dilated cardiomyopathy differs based on diet type. *Journal of Veterinary Cardiology* 21, 1–9. doi: 10.1016/j.jvc.2018.11.002. PMID: 30797439

Anderson, K.L., O'Neill, D.G., Brodbelt, D.C., Church, D.B., Meeson, R.L. *et al.* (2018) Prevalence, duration, and risk factors for appendicular osteoarthritis in a UK dog population under primary veterinary care. *Scientific Reports* 8, 5641. doi: 10.1038/s41598-018-23940-z

Anderson, K.L., Zulch, H., O'Neill, D.G., Meeson, R.L. and Collins L.M. (2020) Risk factors for canine osteoarthritis and its predisposing arthropathies: a systematic review. *Frontiers in Veterinary Science* 7, 220. doi: 10.3389/fvets.2020.00220

Arenas-Montes, J., Perez-Martinez, P., Vals-Delgado, C., Romero-Cabrera, J.L., Cardelo, M.P. *et al.* (2021) Owning a pet is associated with changes in the composition of gut microbiota and could influence the risk of metabolic disorders in humans. *Animals* 11, 2347. doi: org/10.3390/ani11082347

Arkow, P. (1994) Child abuse, animal abuse and the veterinarian. *Journal of the American Veterinary Medical Association* 204, 1004–1007.

ASH (2015) *Smoke legislation: the Health Act 2006.* Action on Smoking and Health. Available at: https://ash.org.uk/wp-content/uploads/2019/10/Smokefree-Legislation.pdf (accessed November 2021).

Azad, M.B., Konya, T., Maughan, H., Guttman, D.S., Field, C.J. *et al.* (2013) Infant gut microbiota and the hygiene hypothesis of allergic disease: impact of household pets and siblings on microbiota composition and diversity. *Allergy, Asthma & Clinical Immunology* 9, 15.

Barbour, K.E., Helmick, C.G., Boring, M. and Brady, T.J. (2017) Vital signs: prevalence of doctor-diagnosed arthritis and arthritis-attributable activity limitation – United States, 2013–2015. *Morbidity and Mortality Weekly Report* 66(9), 246–253. doi: 10.15585/mmwr.mm6609e1

Bawazeer, S., Watson, D.G. and Knottenbelt, C. (2012) Determination of nicotine exposure in dogs subjected to smoking using methanol extraction of hair followed by hydrophilic interaction chromatography in combination with Fourier transform mass spectrometry. *Talanta* 88, 408–411.

Belshaw, Z., Dean, R. and Asher, L. (2020a) Could it be osteoarthritis? How dog owners and veterinary surgeons describe identifying canine osteoarthritis in a general practice setting. *Preventive Veterinary Medicine* 185, 105198.

Belshaw, Z., Dean, R. and Asher, L. (2020b) 'You can be blind because of loving them so much': the impact on owners in the United Kingdom of living with a dog with osteoarthritis. *BMC Veterinary Research* 16, 190.

Bertone, E.R., Synder, L.A. and Moore, A.S. (2002) Environmental tobacco smoke and risk of malignant lymphoma in pet cats. *American Journal of Epidemiology* 156(3), 268–273.

Bhatnagar, P., Wickramasinghe, K., Wilkins, E. and Townsend, N. (2016) Trends in the epidemiology of cardiovascular disease in the UK. *Heart* 102, 1945–1952. doi: 10.1136/heartjnl-2016-309573

The British Geriatric Society (2015) Musculoskeletal conditions: the case for better data. Available at: https://www.bgs.org.uk/blog/musculoskeletal-conditions-the-case-for-better-data (accessed October 2021).

BVA (2019) *One Health in Action. British Veterinary Association Report*, November 2019. Available at: https://www.bva.co.uk/media/3145/bva_one_health_in_action_report_nov_2019.pdf (accessed August 2022).

Byers, C.G. and Dhupa, N. (2005) Feline bronchial asthma: pathophysiology and diagnosis. *Compendium of Continuing Education for Practising Veterinarians* 27(6), 418–425.

CAADA (2014) *In plain sight: effective help for children exposed to domestic abuse* (policy report). Co-ordinated Action Against Domestic Abuse, CAADA Insight 2. available at: https://safelives.org.uk/node/450 (accessed January 2022).

CAM (2021) *Canine arthritis management*. Available at: https://caninearthritis.co.uk/ (accessed November 2021)

Canola, R., Sousa, M., Braz, J., Restan, W., Yamada, D. *et al.* (2018) Cardiorespiratory evaluation of brachycephalic syndrome in dogs. *Pesquisa Veterinária Brasileira* 38(60), 1130–1136.

CDC (2021) *General information about secondhand smoke*. Centers for Disease Control and Prevention. Available at: https://www.cdc.gov/tobacco/data_statistics/fact_sheets/secondhand_smoke/general_facts/index.htm (accessed October 2021)

Chandler, M., Cunningham, S., Lund, E.M., Khanna, C., Naramore, R. *et al.* (2017) Obesity associated comorbidities in people and companion animals: a One Health perspective. *Journal of Comparative Pathology* 156(4), 296–309.

Charles, N. and Davies, C.A. (2008) My family and other animals: pets as kin. *Sociological Research Online* 13(4), 13–26.

Collins. S. (2016) *Heart disease in cats: identifying and managing feline heart disease in practice*. Available at: https://www.veterinary-practice.com/article/heart-disease-in-cats-identifying-and-managing-feline-heart-disease-in-practice (accessed July 2022).

Courcier, E.A., Thomson, R.M., Mellor, D.J. and Yam, P.S. (2010) An epidemiological study of environmental factors associated with canine obesity. *Journal of Small Animal Practice* 51(7), 362–367.

Courcier, E.A., Mellor, D.J. and Thomson, R.M. (2011) A cross sectional study of the prevalence and risk factors for owner misperception of canine body shape in first opinion practice in Glasgow. *Preventive Veterinary Medicine*. 102(1): 66–74.

Dogs Trust (2022) *Hope Project*. Available at: www.dogstrust.org.uk/help-advice/hope-project-freedom-project/hope-project (accessed July 2022).

EarthDay (2020) *Tiny but deadly: cigarette butts are the most commonly polluted plastic*. Available at: https://www.earthday.org/tiny-but-deadly-cigarette-butts-are-the-most-commonly-polluted-plastic/ (accessed March 2022).

Farnworth, M., Packer, R., Sordo, L., Chen, R., Caney, S. and Gunn-Moore, D. (2018) In the eye of the beholder: owner preferences for variations in cats' appearances with specific focus on skull morphology. *Animals* 8(2), E30. doi: 10.3390/ani8020030

Freid, K.J., Freeman, L.M., Rush, J.E., Cunningham, S.M., Davis, M.S. *et al.* (2021) Retrospective study of dilated cardiomyopathy in dogs. *Journal of Veterinary Internal Medicine*. 35(1), 58–67. doi: 10.1111/jvim.15972

German, A.J. (2015) Style over substance: what can parenting styles tell us about ownership styles and obesity in companion animals? *British Journal of Nutrition* 113, S72–S77. doi: 10.1017/S0007114514002335

Häsler, B., Cornelsen, L., Bennani, H. and Rushton, J. (2014) A review of the metrics for One Health benefits. *Revue scientifique et technique* 33, 453–464.

Hayes, H.M., Wilson, G.P. and Fraumeni, J.F. (1982) Carcinoma of the nasal cavity and paranasal sinuses in dogs: descriptive epidemiology. *Cornell Veterinarian* 72, 168–179.

Holmes, K.L., Morris, P.J., Abdulla, Z., Hackett, R. and Rawlings, J.M. (2007) Risk factors associated with excess body weight in dogs in the UK. *Journal of Animal Physiology and Animal Nutrition* 91, 166–167.

Ka, D., Marignac, G., Desquilbet, L., Freyburger, L., Hubert, B. *et al.* (2014) Association between passive smoking and atopic dermatitis in dogs. *Food and Chemical Toxicology* 66, 329–333.

Kienzle, E. and Bergler, R. (2006) Human–animal relationship of owners of normal and overweight cats. *The Journal of Nutrition* 136(7 Suppl.), 1947S–1950S.

Kienzle, E., Bergler, R. and Mandernach, A. (1998) Comparison of the feeding behavior and the human–animal relationship in owners of normal and obese dogs. *The Journal of Nutrition* 128(12 suppl.), 2779S–2782S.

Kim, S.Y., Sim, S. and Choi, H.G. (2017) Atopic dermatitis is associated with active and passive cigarette smoking in adolescents. *PLoS ONE* 12(11), e0187453.

Kramer, U., Lemmen, C.H., Behrendt, H., Link, E., Schafer, T. *et al.* (2004) The effect of environmental tobacco smoke on eczema and allergic sensitization in children. *The British Journal of Dermatology* 150(1), 111–118.

Lascelles, B.D., Hansen, B.D., Roe, S., DePuy, V., Thomson, A. *et al.* (2007) Evaluation of client-specific outcome measures and activity monitoring to measure pain relief in cats with osteoarthritis. *Journal of Veterinary Internal Medicine* 21(3), 410–416. doi: 10.1892/0891-6640(2007)21[410: eocoma]2.0.co;2

Lascelles, B., Henry, J., Robertson, I., Sumrell, A.T., Simpson, W. *et al.* (2010) Cross-sectional study of the prevalence of radiographic degenerative joint disease in domesticated cats. *Veterinary Surgery* 39, 535–544.

Levine, G.N., Allen, K., Braun, L.T., Christian, H.E., Friedmann, E. *et al.* (2013) Pet ownership and cardiovascular risk: a scientific statement from the American Heart Association. *Circulation* 127, 2353–2363.

Maranda, L. and Gupta, O.T. (2016) Association between responsible pet ownership and glycemic control in youths with type 1 diabetes. *PLoS ONE* 11(4), e0152332.

Matthews, K., Kronen, P.W., Lascelles, D., Nolan, A., Roberton, S. *et al.* (2014) Guidelines for recognition, assessment and treatment of pain. *Journal of Small Animal Practice* 55(6), E10–68.

McReynolds, T. (2019) *Flame retardant found in upholstered furniture may cause hyperthyroidism in cats.* AAHA Publications, American Animal Hospital Association. Available at: https://www.aaha.org/publications/newstat/articles/2019-08/flame-retardant-found-in-upholstered-furniture-may-cause-hyperthyroidism-in-cats/ (accessed December 2021).

Meeson, R.L., Todhunter, R., Blunn, G., Nuki, G. and Pitsillides, A.A. (2019) Spontaneous dog osteoarthritis — a One Medicine vision. *Nature Reviews Rheumatology* 15, 273–287. doi: 10.1038/s41584-019-0202-1

Mubanga, M., Byberg, L., Nowak, C., Egenvall, A., Jagnusson, P.K. *et al.* (2017) Dog ownership and the risk of cardiovascular disease and death – a nationwide co-hort study. *Scientific Reports* 7(1), 15821.

Munro, H.M.C. and Thrusfield, M.V. (2001a) 'Battered Pets': features that raise suspicion of non-accidental injury. *Journal of Small Animal Practice* 42, 218–226.

Munro, H.M.C. and Thrusfield, M.V. (2001b) 'Battered Pets': non-accidental physical injuries found in dogs and cats. *Journal of Small Animal Practice* 42, 279–290.

Munro, H.M.C. and Thrusfield, M.V. (2001c) 'Battered Pets': sexual abuse. *Journal of Small Animal Practice* 42, 333–337.

Munro, H.M.C. and Thrusfield, M.V. (2001d) 'Battered Pets': Munchausen syndrome by proxy (factitious illness by proxy). *Journal of Small Animal Practice* 42, 385–389.

Natterson-Horowitz, B., Desmarchelie, M., Winkler, A. and Carabin, H. (2022) Beyond zoonoses in One Health: non-communicable diseases across the animal kingdom. *Frontiers in Public Health* 9, 807186. doi: 10.3389/fpubh.2021.807186

NCCIH (2022) *Natural doesn't necessarily mean safer, or better.* National Center for Complementary and Integrative Health. Available at: https://www.nccih.nih.gov/health/know-science/natural-doesnt-mean-better (accessed April 2022).

NHS (2021) *Passive smoking.* Available at: https://www.nhs.uk/live-well/quit-smoking/passive-smoking-protect-your-family-and-friends/ (accessed November 2021).

NHS Inform (2020) *Second-hand smoke.* Available at: https://www.nhsinform.scot/healthy-living/stopping-smoking/reasons-to-stop/second-hand-smoke (accessed December 2021).

NHS Inform (2021a) *Chronic pain.* Available at: https://www.nhsinform.scot/illnesses-and-conditions/brain-nerves-and-spinal-cord/chronic-pain (accessed March 2022).

NHS Inform (2021b) *Take it right outside.* Available at: https://www.nhsinform.scot/campaigns/take-it-right-outside (accessed November 2021)

O'Neill, D., Skipper, A., Kadham, J., Church, D., Brodbelt, D. and Packer, R. (2019) Disorders of Bulldogs under primary veterinary care in the UK in 2013. *PLoS ONE* 14(6), e0217928. doi: 10.1371/journal.pone.0217928

O'Neill, D.G., Pegram, C., Crocker, P., Brodbelt, D.C., Church, D.B. and Packer, R.M.A. (2020) Unravelling the health status of brachycephalic dogs in the UK using multivariable analysis. *Scientific Report* 10, 17251.

ONS (2020) *Adult smoking habit in the UK – 2019.* Office for National Statistics. Available at: https://www.ons.gov.uk/peoplepopulationandcommunity/healthandsocialcare/healthandlifeexpectancies/bulletins/adultsmokinghabitsingreatbritain/2019 (accessed December 2021).

Packer, R.M.A., Murphy, D. and Farnworth, M.J. (2017) Purchasing popular pure-breds: investigating the influence of breed-type on the pre-purchase attitudes and behaviour of dog owners. *Animal Welfare* 26(2), 191–201.

Poutasse, C.M., Herbstman, J., Peterson, M.E., Gordon, J., Soboroff, P.H. *et al.* (2019) Silicone pet tags associate tris(1,3-dichloro-2-isopropyl) phosphate exposures with feline hyperthyroidism. *Environmental Science & Technology* 53(15), 9203–9213. doi: 10.1021/acs.est.9b02226

RCVS (2021) *Code of Professional Conduct for Veterinary Nurses.* Royal College of Veterinary Surgeons. Available at: https://www.rcvs.org.uk/setting-standards/

advice-and-guidance/code-of-professional-conduct-for-veterinary-nurses/ (accessed December 2021)

Reif, J.S., Bruns, C. and Lower, K.S. (1998) Cancer of the nasal cavity and paranasal sinuses and exposure to environmental tobacco smoke in pet dogs. *American Journal of Epidemiology* 147(5), 488–492.

Reinero, C.R., DeClue, A.E. and Rabinowitz, P. (2009) Asthma in humans and cats: is there a common sensitivity to aeroallegens in shared environments? *American Journal of Epidemiology and Environmental Research* 109 (5), 634–640.

Rijnberk, A.S., Kooistra, H.S. and Mol, J.A. (2003) Endocrine diseases in dogs and cats: similarities and differences with endocrine diseases in humans. *Growth Hormone & IGF Research* 13 (Suppl.), S158–S164. doi: 10.1016/S1096-6374(03)00076-5

RSPCA (2019) *Does cigarette smoke affect our pets?* Royal Society for the Prevention of Cruelty to Animals. Available at: https://kb.rspca.org.au/knowledge-base/does-cigarette-smoke-affect-pets/ (accessed January 2022).

RVC (2021) *Understanding brachycephalic ownership. Royal Veterinary College.* Available at: https://www.rvc.ac.uk/research/focus/brachycephaly/latest-research/projects/understanding-brachycephalic-ownership (accessed December 2021).

Safiri, S., Kolahi, A.A., Smith, E., Hill, C., Bettampadi, D. *et al.* (2020) Global, regional and national burden of osteoarthritis 1990–2017: a systematic analysis of the Global Burden of Disease Study 2017. *Annals of the Rheumatic Diseases* 79(6), 819-828.

Schreiner, P.J. (2016) Emerging cardiovascular risk research: impact of pets on cardiovascular risk prevention. *Current Cardiovascular Risk Reports* 10(2), 8.

Slingerland, L., Hazelwinkle, H., Meij, B., Pica, P. and Voorhout, G. (2011) Cross-sectional study of the prevalence and clinical features of osteoarthritis in 100 cats. *Veterinary Journal* 187, 304–309.

Snyder, L.A., Bertone, E.R, Jakowski, R.M., Dooner, M.S., Jennings-Ritchie, J. and Moore, A.S. (2004) p53 expression and environmental tobacco smoke exposure in feline oral squamous cell carcinoma. *Veterinary Pathology* 41(3), 209–240.

Social Mobility Commission (2016) *Socio-economic influences on children's life chances.* Available at: https://www.gov.uk/government/news/socio-economic-influences-on-childrens-life-chances (accessed December 2021)

Statista (2021) *Share of households owning a pet in the United Kingdom (UK) from 2011/12 to 2020/21.* Statista Research Department. Available at: https://www.statista.com/statistics/308235/estimated-pet-ownership-in-the-united-kingdom-uk/ (accessed December 2021).

Tobacco Free Life (2016) *Smoking environmental risks.* Available at: https://tobacofreelife.org/why-quit-smoking/smoking-effects/smoking-environmental-risks/ (accessed January 2020).

Tun, H.M., Konya, T., Takaro, T.K., Brook, J.R., Chari, R. *et al.* (2017) Exposure to household furry pets influences the gut microbiota of infant at 3–4 months following various birth scenarios. *Microbiome* 5(1), 40.

WHO (2021) *Noncommunicable diseases.* World Health Organization. Available at: https://www.who.int/news-room/fact-sheets/detail/noncommunicable-diseases (accessed July 2022).

Williams, A.C.C. (2019) Persistence of pain in humans and other mammals. *Philosophical Transactions of the Royal Society of London. Series B, Biological Sciences* 374(1785), 20190276. doi: 10.1098/rstb.2019.0276

Women's Aid (2021) *What is domestic abuse?* Available at: https://www.womensaid. org.uk/information-support/what-is-domestic-abuse/ (accessed December 2021).

Yeh, T.L., Lei, W.T., Liu, S.J. and Chien, K.L. (2019) A modest protective association between pet ownership and cardiovascular diseases: a systematic review and meta-analysis. *PLoS ONE* 14(5), e0216231.

Communicable Diseases

5

Emi N. Barker[1]* and Marta Costa[2]

[1]*Langford Vets, University of Bristol, UK;* [2]*Bristol Veterinary School, University of Bristol, UK*

Key points

- The definition of communicable disease, how it is transmitted and examples of causal agents
- Examples of emerging and zoonotic diseases and how these can be mitigated in the veterinary setting
- The influence of veterinary healthcare on communicable disease

5.1   Definition of Communicable Disease

Communicable diseases are those that can be transmitted or 'communicated' from one individual to another – either directly or near-directly (also termed contagious disease) or indirectly, e.g. via an intermediate organism or fomite (Fig. 5.1). Communicable diseases are also considered 'infectious', although not every infectious disease is considered communicable. While many infectious diseases are caused by obligate infectious agents (in that these agents require a host for replication and onwards transmission), some infectious diseases are caused by opportunists, typically environmental, commensal, or symbiotic organisms, that access privileged sites; these are not considered communicable.

Environmental microorganisms replicate outside of a potential host, while both commensal and symbiotic microorganisms replicate within specific host sites (e.g. mucosal surface or epithelial surface, such as the gastrointestinal tract or skin) and under normal conditions are either neutral or beneficial to the host. Examples of opportunistic infection include: sinonasal aspergillosis in dogs (infectious agent: fungus, *Aspergillus fumigatus*; source of infection: environmental; site: sinonasal mucosa; exposure: via inhalation of spores); tetanus in multiple species (infectious agent: bacterium, *Clostridium tetani*; source of infection: environmental; site: (deep/penetrating) wounds,

Email: Emi.barker@bristol.ac.uk

© CAB International 2023. *One Health for Veterinary Nurses and Technicians* (eds R. Jones and A. Jeffery)
DOI: 10.1079/9781789249477.0005

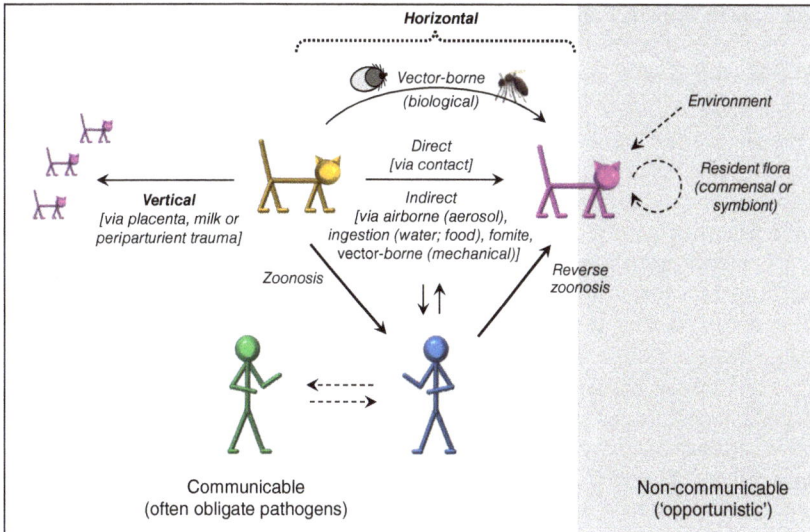

Fig. 5.1. Source of the pathogens causing infectious disease. The source determines whether the disease is communicable or (generally) non-communicable. Different routes of transmission are possible and are important to consider when determining risk and methods to limit spread.

rarely post-surgical; exposure: tissue inoculation of spores, with subsequent replication and release of toxin); cat bite abscesses (infectious agent: bacterium such as *Pasteurella multocida*; site: subcutaneous; exposure: bacteria from teeth/mouth are inoculated into tissue during biting); and surgical site infection (infectious agent: bacterium such as *Staphylococcus pseudintermedius*; site: surgical; exposure: bacteria from skin surface are permitted access to subcutaneous and deeper tissues following interruption of epithelial barrier or iatrogenic inoculation).

The line between obligate infectious agent and opportunist can be blurred. While most cases of lower urinary tract infection are opportunistic (infectious agent: usually bacteria such as *Escherichia coli* or *Staphylococcus* spp., rarely fungi; source of infection: faecal or cutaneous flora; site: bladder; exposure: usually ascending infection from the external genitalia, occasionally iatrogenic following urinary catheterization), uropathogenic bacteria with increased propensity to cause disease (i.e. virulence factors) can be transmitted between individuals and between species resulting in communicable urinary tract infection and outbreaks of disease (e.g. some strains of enteroaggregative *Escherichia coli*). Similarly, commensal flora can also be 'shared' or communicated between individuals, including ones with potentially significant virulence factors or antimicrobial resistance mechanism such as methicillin-resistance (e.g. methicillin-resistant *Staph. pseudintermedius*, MRSP).

5.2 The Agents of Communicable Disease

A wide variety of agents can cause disease (Fig. 5.2). They can be transmitted in one or more different ways (Figs 5.1 and 5.2 and section 5.3) and can enter the body via different routes. Pathogens cause disease either directly (i.e. during replication or via toxins production) or indirectly (i.e. manifestation of the host response to pathogen presence) or via a combination of both mechanisms. Therefore, individual response to infection with pathogens can be highly variable.

To complicate matters, the definitions of 'infectious disease' and 'pathogen' can vary between authors. Some prefer a simplistic definition: 'infectious diseases are caused by pathogenic organisms', i.e. infection with a smaller living entity distinct from the host that can cause damage to the host. This definition of pathogenic organisms will encompass species of bacteria, protozoa, moulds, algae, fungi, etc. However, viruses clearly cause many infectious diseases yet are considered by many not to be organisms, being entirely reliant on host cell machinery for metabolism and ultimately replication. Other pathogens that cannot be pigeon-holed into this simple definition include prions (i.e. misfolded proteins; the causative agents of transmissible spongiform encephalopathies) and transmissible cancers (i.e. living clonal cells that are genetically distinct from the 'infected' host animal, but can develop into tumours and be transmitted between individuals). Some authors define pathogens as being microscopic, such that larger agents of infectious disease such as

Pathogen	Routes of transmission between individuals	Point of entry into the body
Bacteria	Airborne (e.g. cough, sneeze, aerosol)	Skin – intact or broken
Fungi		Mucous membranes (ocular, oral, urogenital)
Viruses	Bodily fluids or tissue (e.g. blood, urine, semen, milk)	
Algae		Respiratory tract (i.e. inhalation)
	Contaminated environment (e.g. air, water, hard surfaces)	
Oomycete		Gastrointestinal tract (i.e. ingestion)
Helminth	Contaminated object (i.e. fomite)	
Protozoa		Injection (e.g. iatrogenic; insect/tick bites; aggressive interaction)
	Contaminated organisms (i.e. mechanical vector)	
Prions		
Neoplastic cells		Transplacental
	Infected organisms – biological vector or intermediate host	

Fig. 5.2. List of pathogen types that have been associated with communicable diseases, the various routes of transmission between individuals, and the point of entry into the body.

helminths (i.e. worms capable of causing disease) are considered separately as parasites alongside other organisms such as arthropods (i.e. ticks, biting flies, fleas).

Table 5.1 gives selected examples of common infectious diseases.

Table 5.1. Selected examples of common infectious, often communicable, diseases from the broad categories given in Fig. 5.2 as well as additional examples of those with zoonotic potential. (Please note that this list is not exhaustive.)

Table 5.1a Viruses

Examples of diseases and their causative agents	Examples with zoonotic potential

RNA viruses

Canine distemper virus	**Hantavirus**
A paramyxovirus related to the measles virus in humans. It is a significant cause of morbidity and mortality where vaccination is not practised. It can infect a wide variety of other species, including giant pandas (causing high mortality) and large cats (often subclinical).	Transmitted from rodents (where it is subclinical) to humans via inhalation of infectious material (urine, saliva, faeces). Can cause haemorrhagic fever with renal syndrome, with the potential to progress to death. One study showed nearly 40% of pet rat owners had evidence of exposure.
Feline calicivirus (FCV)	**Rabies (and other lyssaviruses)**
One of the causative agents of 'cat flu' and the agent of 'FCV-associated virulent systemic disease'.	Transmitted from other mammals to humans via saliva contact with mucous membranes or bite wounds.
Bovine viral diarrhoea virus	It causes fatal encephalomyelitis.
A pestivirus that causes bovine viral diarrhoea or mucosal disease (BVD-MD), the latter occurring due to intrauterine infection. It has a significant financial impact on the livestock industry.	It causes over 50,000 deaths per year, often in developing countries.
	West Nile virus
Feline infectious peritonitis virus	A flavivirus transmitted by mosquitoes. The primary hosts are birds. In
An alpha coronavirus that causes severe systemic disease (fatal if not treated with antivirals). It arises in individual cats from the frequently benign feline enteric coronavirus.	humans it can cause a wide range of presentations from flu-like symptoms to meningitis and encephalitis. Horses can be similarly affected. Infected dogs and cats rarely show clinical signs.

Retroviruses (specialist RNA viruses that can integrate within the host genome)

Feline leukaemia virus (FeLV)	**Simian immunodeficiency virus (SIV-1)**
An oncovirus that can cause a wide variety of haematological malignancies in cats.	SIV-1 is thought to have 'jumped species' from primates to humans, resulting in human immunodeficiency
Feline immunodeficiency virus (FIV)	virus (HIV). Between humans HIV transmission can be venereal, vertical,
A lentivirus that can cause immunosuppression in cats. It is in the same genus as SIV and HIV but is not zoonotic.	or iatrogenic (e.g. transfusion of contaminated blood products or re-use of contaminated equipment).

Continued

Table 5.1a Continued.

Examples of diseases and their causative agents	Examples with zoonotic potential
DNA viruses **Canine and feline parvoviruses** The causative agents of canine parvoviral enteritis and feline infectious enteritis, respectively. A significant cause of morbidity and mortality in both species where vaccination is not practised. **Feline herpesvirus** One of the causative agents of 'cat flu'. A common cause of ocular and respiratory disease in cats. Infection typically leads to a chronic carrier state with occasional recrudescence.	**B-virus (Macacine alphaherpesvirus 1)** In rhesus monkeys it causes subclinical or cold-sore-like disease, while in humans it causes severe encephalitis with high mortality. Transmission is in bodily fluids via contact with mucous membranes or bite wounds. **Cowpox virus** (related to smallpox virus and monkeypox virus) Transmitted to humans most often from infected cats, that acquire the infection from rodents via bites. Affected cats are typically presented for veterinary care with crusting dermatological lesions on the head, neck and feet, or with respiratory tract signs. In humans it usually causes cutaneous pustular lesions.

Table 5.1b Bacteria

Examples of diseases and their causative agents	Examples with zoonotic potential
Members of the Proteobacteria phylum (including *Escherichia coli, Campylobacter* spp., *Salmonella* spp., *Yersinia pestis, Vibrio cholerae*) These are common causes of both opportunistic and communicable disease. Many of the members of this group are facultative anaerobes, which lends them to survival within both the gastrointestinal tract of mammals (and shedding in faeces) as well as in moist environments outside the host, such as watercourses. They can be commensals in some mammals and pathogenic in others, depending on host susceptibility and virulence of bacterial strain. For example, salmonellosis in cats (causing diarrhoea, pyrexia and lethargy) is sometimes termed 'songbird fever' as it is more frequently seen in avid hunters – frequently following an outbreak of salmonellosis in birds.	Many Proteobacteria can cause food-borne gastroenteritis in humans as well as other mammals (e.g. cholera, salmonellosis, campylobacteriosis). These organisms can also cause sepsis if there is systemic spread. Transmission follows ingestion of contaminated food or water, or through poor hygiene when handling infectious material (e.g. faeces, raw meat). ***Mycobacterium tuberculosis* complex (inc. *M. tuberculosis, M. bovis,* and *M. microti*)** *Mycobacterium tuberculosis* is the causative agent of human tuberculosis and can be a reverse zoonosis to household pets. *Mycobacterium bovis* is the causative agent of bovine tuberculosis (bTB) but can infect a wide variety of species.

Continued

Table 5.1b Continued.

Examples of diseases and their causative agents	Examples with zoonotic potential
Arthropod vector-borne obligate intracellular pathogens *Ehrlichia* spp., *Anaplasma* spp., *Rickettsia* spp. and *Borrelia burgdorferi* These cause disease because of destruction of infected cells and via the induction of secondary immune-mediated inflammation (e.g. thrombocytopenia associated with ehrlichiosis due to *Ehrlichia canis* in dogs). Both Rocky Mountain spotted fever, caused by *Rickettsia rickettsii*, and Lyme disease, caused by *B. burgdorferi*, can occur in humans and dogs. Transmission is via haematophagous activity of ticks, although tick attachment is frequently missed. Dogs can act as sentinels of disease, a mechanical vector for infected ticks, and as a source of infection (i.e. ticks feeding consecutively on an infected dog and then their owner). **Chlamydia felis** Another obligate intracellular pathogen, and cause of infectious conjunctivitis in cats. **Mycoplasma spp.** Various mycoplasmas infect mucosal surfaces (e.g. *Mycoplasma cynos* causing cough in the dog; *Mycoplasma felis* causing conjunctivitis in the cat; *Mycoplasma mycoides* causing bronchopneumonia in cattle), joint surfaces (e.g. *Mycoplasma synoviae* in poultry and *Mycoplasma hyosynoviae* in swine causing lameness), and red blood cells (e.g. *Mycoplasma suis* in pigs and *Mycoplasma haemofelis* in cats causing anaemia). Their reduced genome means that cultivation in vitro is often difficult and slow, to impossible. As they lack a cell wall, they are intrinsically resistant to some antimicrobials (e.g. penicillins).	Bacteria are transmitted to and between humans, companion animals (including dogs and cats), livestock and wildlife through contaminated meat, unpasteurized milk, sputum and urine. Clinical signs cannot be used to distinguish infecting species. Disease is chronic, potentially life-threatening and difficult to treat. **Staph. aureus and Staph. pseudintermedius** Common causes of opportunistic infections, as well as being reverse zoonoses and zoonoses, respectively. They are common causes of nosocomial infection in human and veterinary healthcare settings, respectively, and cause particular concern where there is multi-drug resistance (i.e. MRSA or MRSP). **Yersinia pestis** The causative agent of the bubonic plague, causes bacteraemia and is transmitted via the haematophagous activity of fleas (i.e. arthropod vector). Transmission to humans is primarily from rats, but cats (and rabbits and dogs) can also be a source. **Chlamydia psittaci** The causative agent of psittacosis ('parrot fever'), a potentially fatal disease in humans. Transmission is vial inhalation of infectious material, often in the form of dried faeces while cleaning cages. Although members of the psittacine family (which includes budgerigars) are most frequently implicated, turkeys and pigeons have also been implicated in some cases.

Continued

Table 5.1b Continued.

Examples of diseases and their causative agents	Examples with zoonotic potential
	Leptospira interrogans
	Various members of the group (which includes serovar *icterohaemorrhagiae*, the causative agent of Weil's disease) cause disease in humans. Transmission usually follows exposure of mucosal surfaces (or broken skin) to infected urine, via ingestion or splashing. A wide variety of mammalian species, including the dog, can carry infection and spread disease. Vaccination in dogs can reduce this risk.

Table 5.1c Helminths (i.e. parasitic worms – including nematodes, trematodes and cestodes)

Examples of diseases and their causative agents	Examples with zoonotic potential
Dirofilaria immitis	***Echinococcus granulosus***
The cause of canine heartworm. It is transmitted by mosquitos, and its distribution is limited by this vector.	The cause of hydatid disease in humans (as an aberrant intermediate host). Dogs are the definitive host for the adult tapeworms (< 6 mm length) – with eggs shed in faeces.
Dipylidium caninum	**Ocular and visceral larval migrans**
The canine and feline tapeworm. It is spread by fleas, so when found multimodal anti-parasitic treatment is indicated.	Can occur in humans following the ingestion of nematodes, including *Toxocara canis*, *Toxocara cati* and *Ascaris suum*.

5.3 Transmission

Pathogen transmission can be described in a variety of ways (Figs 5.1 and 5.2 and Tables 5.2a–c).

Many pathogens can be transmitted via more than one route, with pathogen factors (e.g. physical size; capacity for environmental survival; bodily fluids/tissue in which the pathogen is contained and shed; presence of life cycle

Table 5.1d Protozoa

Examples of diseases and their causative agents	Examples with zoonotic potential
Leishmania infantum The causative agent of leishmaniasis in Europe. It is a frequent cause of chronic disease (crusting dermatopathy, polyarthritis, kidney disease) in dogs originating from Southern European countries. Horizontal transmission in the absence of the usual sandfly vector and vertical transmission are both possible. In areas where the sandfly vector is present, dogs act as sentinels of disease. Vaccination reduces the risk of disease.	**_Toxoplasma gondii_** The definitive host is the cat, which sheds oocysts in faeces resulting in environmental contamination and rarely develops clinical disease (toxoplasmosis). Toxoplasmosis in other mammalian intermediate hosts (including humans, dogs and sheep) follows accidental ingestion, and can manifest as systemic inflammation, encephalitis and abortion. Infection in humans usually follows ingestion of contaminated meat or soil (from gardening) and rarely follows direct handling of cat litter (oocysts only become infective > 24 h after being passed in faeces).

Table 5.1e Fungal (moulds and yeasts)

Examples of diseases and their causative agents	Examples with zoonotic potential
Aspergillus fumigatus The causative agent of sinonasal aspergillosis in the dog. Fungal plaques on the respiratory mucosa cause an intense inflammatory response resulting in tissue destruction (initially turbinate loss and epistaxis, progressing to destruction of the cribriform plate). **_Malassezia pachydermatis_** The cause of Malassezia dermatitis in dogs. It is usually secondary to another problem, such as atopy.	**_Sporothrix schenckii_** The causative agent of sporotrichosis in cats and dogs. It typically causes cutaneous granulomas. Although zoonotic transmission from dogs is rare, it is not uncommon from cats. Most frequently reported in animals from South America and Africa, with increased movement of cats (and dogs) from this could be an emerging concern. **Fungal skin infection** (dermatophytosis, e.g. _Trichophyton_ spp., _Microsporum_ spp., and _Epidermophyton_ spp.) Not uncommon in young or immunocompromised animals. Many have zoonotic potential, and gloves should be worn when handling possible cases, with efforts made to reduce the risk of aerosolization.

Table 5.1f Algae

Examples of diseases and their causative agents	Examples with zoonotic potential
***Prototheca* spp.** The cause of protothecosis in dogs (and humans). A rare algal infection associated with severe granulomatous change often involving the gastrointestinal tract, as well as ocular, cutaneous and disseminated forms. Attempted treatment has not been successful.	Protothecosis in companion animals is thought to be of low risk for zoonotic transmission to humans.

Table 5.1g Oomycetes

Examples of diseases and their causative agents	Examples with zoonotic potential
Pythium insidiosum The cause of pythiosis in horses, dogs and (rarely) cats, where granulomatous or ulcerative lesions form. It does not appear to be transmissible. ***Lagenidium* spp.** The cause of lagenidiosis in dogs, where granulomatous or ulcerative lesions form. It does not appear to be transmissible.	None

Table 5.1h Prions

Examples of diseases and their causative agents	Examples with zoonotic potential
Transmissible spongiform encephalopathies Including Scrapie in sheep, Chronic Wasting Disease in deer, Bovine Spongiform Encephalopathy (BSE) in cattle, and Creutzfeldt–Jakob Disease in humans.	Transmission of bovine spongiform encephalopathy-associated prions to humans, primarily through ingestion of beef offal, can result in variant Creutzfeldt–Jakob disease.

Table 5.1i Neoplastic cells

Examples of diseases and their causative agents	Examples with zoonotic potential
The three forms described to date are canine transmissible venereal tumour (TVT), devil facial tumour disease in Tasmanian devils, and contagious reticulum cell sarcoma in Syrian hamsters (experimental).	None

stages requiring alternative hosts), host factors (e.g. immunity; vaccination status; carrier status; age; concurrent disease) and environmental factors (e.g. presence of vector; temperature; density of housing; contact with wildlife reservoirs) influencing the route via which transmission is most likely to occur. For example, canine parvovirus is a non-enveloped virus shed in faeces with the ability to remain infective in the environment for many months; while, following infection (or successful immunization), duration of sterile immunity (i.e. where infection and transmission are completely prevented by host immunity) is long-lived. This means that, as well as direct dog-to-dog faeco-oral transmission from a newly infected case, indirect transmission can occur within a kennel or veterinary hospital on fomites (e.g. bedding, grooming brushes, leads and collars), on people (e.g. moving between patients without cleaning hands), following aerosolization (e.g. when spraying down dirty kennels), while infection from a contaminated environment (e.g. the local dog park) plays a significant role in disease persistence within a population. In contrast, *Ehrlichia canis* is a blood-borne bacterium that does not survive outside the dog or tick (biological vector); while, following clinical disease, subclinical infection is potentially lifelong and vaccination is not available. This means that the distribution of the primary arthropod vector, brown dog tick *Rhipicephalus sanguineus*, is important in environmental persistence and spread, while direct dog-to-dog transmission requires exchange of blood (e.g. blood transfusion; aggressive interactions).

5.4   Emerging and Re-emerging Diseases

Some communicable diseases are endemic within a population. This means that they have been present over an extended time period and are seen frequently. Where it is possible to prevent their transmission, through either vaccination or hygiene measurements, it is possible to decrease their prevalence or even eradicate them (e.g. smallpox in humans and rinderpest in ruminants). Campaigns for vaccination (e.g. rabies) can have a significant impact on preventing both animal and human disease. Increased uptake of vaccination results in lower

Table 5.2a Pathogen transmission: direct versus indirect.

Direct	Indirect
Contact between individuals results in pathogen transmission, often within bodily fluids or tissue	Pathogens are spread via **environmental contamination** (of air, water and hard surfaces), **droplets** (aerosolized bodily fluids containing pathogens), **fomites** (inanimate objects) and **vectors** (other living organisms)

Table 5.2b Categorization of direct transmission according to relationship between donor and recipient.

Transmission type	Definition and comments
Vertical	Where pathogens are transmitted from mother to offspring. A side effect of the hormonal changes that occur during pregnancy is immunosuppression, which increases the likelihood of infection recrudescence and transmission (examples include protozoal parasite *Neospora caninum* and hookworm *Ancylostoma caninum* in dogs). Transmission can occur *in utero*, during parturition, or post-partum, through intimate contact and ingestion of bodily fluids including blood, products of parturition, and milk
Horizontal	Where pathogens are transmitted between peers (i.e. not associated with pregnancy or perinatal period)
Venereal	A special form of horizontal transmission, where pathogens are transmitted during coitus (examples include brucellosis in livestock and dogs; immunodeficiency viruses in cats and humans; and TVT in dogs)

Table 5.2c Biological, mechanical and iatrogenic transmission. Biological vector-borne transmission categorized according to the role the vector plays in the pathogen's biology. Amplification may occur within this vector, and the vector is often specific for the pathogens (for example, the *Phlebotomus* spp., sandfly, in the transmission of *Leishmainia infantum* between humans, dogs and other species).

Type of host	Comments
Biological: Intermediate (secondary) host	Time spent in this host is required for the pathogen to progress through a non-sexual life stage or stages. Asexual amplification may occur. For example, molluscs are intermediate hosts for *Angiostrongylus vasorum* larvae

Continued

Table 5.2c Continued.

Type of host	Comments
Biological: Paratenic (transport) host	Time spent in this host is *not required* for the pathogen to progress through a life stage; however, the pathogen can be maintained in this host or be more likely to be transmitted to the definitive host. For example, frogs are intermediate hosts for *A. vasorum* larvae
Biological: Definitive (primary or final) host	Time spent in this host is required for the pathogen to progress through a sexual life stage. For example, dogs (and other canids, including foxes) are the definitive host for *A. vasorum*. However, mammals are not always the definitive host; mosquitoes are definitive hosts for *Plasmodium* spp., the causative agent of malaria
Mechanical	Where the pathogen is spread via a non-specific intermediary species that plays no role in the life cycle of the pathogen. For example, transmission of feline calicivirus from one cat to another on unwashed human hands
Iatrogenic	Transmission may also be iatrogenic, although rarely maliciously so, via the administration of infected blood products (e.g. haemoplasma infection in cats and babesiosis in dogs) or use of contaminated surgical instruments (e.g. bTB in cats)

levels of the clinical disease they protect against, particularly where 'herd immunity' is achieved.

Re-emerging diseases are those that reappear after a period of absence or are seen infrequently within a population. This can happen, for example, when societal memory of the impact of these infectious agents wanes and consequently the desire to vaccinate. Infectious disease may also re-emerge within a population as the antigenicity of a pathogen diverges from that of the previously circulating strains, such as inadequate immunity exists to prevent spread. For example, parvovirosis can result in life-threatening haemorrhagic gastroenteritis in dogs; however, this is infrequently seen where there is high uptake of vaccination. Failure to vaccinate and loss of herd immunity results in occasional outbreaks. In addition, different strains of the canine parvovirus have arisen over time, resulting in breakthrough infection in vaccinated dogs. Vaccine manufacturers respond to this by adjusting the vaccine strain accordingly.

For some diseases, environmental changes that impact on the geographical distribution of the vector or wildlife reservoir will also impact on the distribution of the pathogen. For example, incidence of bubonic plague in humans increases as do rodent numbers, their primary host (Table 5.1). Another example is canine angiostrongylosis. Over time the distribution of clinical cases has become more widespread and extended further north within Europe. This northern progression is thought to reflect: (i) increased survival of the intermediate hosts (small molluscs) due to increased environmental temperatures alongside increased water availability; (ii) an increased rate of progression from the shed (L1) to the infective (L3) larval forms within the intermediate host at increased environmental temperatures; (iii) an increased prevalence of urban sylvatic populations that are reservoirs of infection; and (iv) increased movement of dogs within and between countries.

Emerging communicable diseases are commonly defined as outbreaks of previously unknown diseases (e.g. by crossing species, or adaptation to a new host, such as with COVID-19), known diseases which have rapidly increased in incidence or geographical range, or persistence of new diseases that cannot be controlled. Increased travel-related disease, incursions into wildlife habitats and increased close contact within species potentiate the appearance of these diseases. Canine brucellosis is a current example of a disease of increasing concern in some countries in Western Europe and North America, as increased numbers of dogs travel internationally (the UK is a net importer of dogs) and the numbers of diagnosed cases have increased. This is of particular concern as *Brucella canis* is zoonotic and many dogs have subclinical infection, passing the pathogen horizontally and vertically within their household (see section 5.3).

5.5   Zoonoses

5.5.1   Definitions and risk factors

Transmission of organisms capable of causing disease may be within a species or between species (Fig. 5.1). Where this occurs *from non-human animal to human* it is termed a **zoonosis**; and where the direction of travel is *from human to non-human animal* it is termed **reverse zoonosis or zooanthroponosis**. Some examples are given in Table 5.1. Approximately 75% of emerging infectious diseases in humans are believed to be zoonoses, which typically occur at an interface between humans and wild animals.

Zoonoses are more likely to occur where there is increased contact with animals, especially where this contact may be close, aggressive or carry increased risk of trauma, or where the animals are sick or stressed (e.g. reduced environmental resources; anxiety/fear of being handled; overcrowded) and more likely to be shedding infection or have higher infectious loads. For these reasons, pet owners and anyone who works with animals (including livestock workers, zookeepers, abattoir workers and veterinary personnel) are at increased risk. Within the veterinary health setting, the risks of acquiring a zoonosis vary between the different disciplines of small animal, exotic pets/wildlife, equine and farm practice.

Many pet owners are unaware of the potential of, or the risk factors associated with, zoonotic disease. Sometimes this is due to mistaken beliefs, based on inaccurate sources of information. In addition, where the perceived risk is lower, through familiarity or lack of knowledge, fewer precautions may be taken to limit the transmission.

Human and animal factors that increase the risk of zoonotic infection are described in Tables 5.3a and 5.3b, respectively.

Sometimes these risk factors can combine. For example, an immunocompromised person may obtain a pet snake and feed it raw meat.

Diet is a common discussion point in veterinary practice (for veterinary surgeons, veterinary nurses and other support staff). Regardless of personal views, it is important to have a balanced discussion with owners who feed raw meat diets, to understand and respect their beliefs, to identify owner and pet risk factors that might increase their respective risks of disease, to suggest risk mitigation strategies, and to direct them towards reputable sources of information. It is also important, when admitting a pet into a hospital, shelter, or boarding situation, to identify those that are fed raw meat, as this will influence how they are nursed, due to the increased risk of transmission to staff or other animals.

Over the past 10–20 years there has been an increasing trend to feed raw meat diets to dogs, and to a lesser extent cats, with commercially prepared raw diets becoming more widely available. Their selection is not based on financial grounds or convenience and their use is often actively encouraged by breeders, on-line interest groups and a minority of veterinary professionals. Some dogs (e.g. with atopy or dietary sensitivities) anecdotally appear to benefit from such diets, possibly due to them containing a limited number of protein sources, making them relatively hypoallergenic along with increased omega-3 fatty acid content. Many dogs and cats find these diets highly palatable. However, there are risks associated with feeding of raw diets that might not be appreciated by owners. Irrespective of the destination plate, due to how it is processed, raw meat products contain significant numbers of faeces-derived bacteria (often strains of *E. coli* and *Campylobacter* spp. and occasionally *Salmonella* spp. – with the potential to cause 'food-poisoning'). Rarely, feeding of raw meat has been associated with bTB infection in dogs and cats, and *Brucella suis* infection in dogs – both infectious agents of significant zoonotic concern. While most dogs often do not develop disease following ingestion of 'food-poisoning' bacteria, fatal infection can occur. Dogs fed raw meat are more likely to shed bacteria of zoonotic concern and bacteria carrying antimicrobial resistance (AMR) genes, as compared with dogs fed a cooked diet. Owners, in handling the raw meat, the food bowls and their pets, increase their frequency of exposure to these organisms. This risk can be reduced, but not eliminated, by following standard

Table 5.3a Human factors that increase the risk of zoonotic infection.

Human factor	Comments and reasons
Young age	Due to a variety of reasons, including: Reduced risk awareness Reduced hand hygiene Sharing of foodstuffs with animals Reduced immunity
Impaired immune response	Due to a variety of reasons, including: Limited repertoire (the very young) Senile changes (the very old) Presence of concurrent disease (resulting in immunocompromise) Pregnancy Receipt of immunosuppressive medications (e.g. chemotherapeutic agents)
Food	Ingestion of raw or undercooked meat, fish or dairy products, or their inappropriate storage and handling leading to contamination of other foodstuffs
High-risk animal husbandry practices	Examples: Feeding of raw meat (including raw-hide treats) Ownership of some exotic pets (for example, reptiles frequently carry *Salmonella*) Allowing the pet access to the face (e.g. to lick or 'kiss'); and co-sleeping
Increased access to large numbers of animals that may be sick or stressed	Examples: farmer, farmworker, abattoir worker, veterinary staff, breeders, and shelter workers
Increased access to animal faeces	Examples: via gardening, handling of cat litter, and where it has been used as a fertilizer

Table 5.3b Animal factors that increase the risk of zoonotic infection.

Animal factor	Comments and reasons
Young age	A combination of increased stress, overcrowding, and immune-system naivety result in an increased likelihood of infectious disease, increased shedding of pathogens at higher copy numbers, and increased dissemination of pathogens (i.e. they are more likely to have diarrhoea)
Outdoor access and hunting behaviour	
Fearful nature	More likely to have an aggressive interaction with others, including humans
High-risk animal husbandry practices	Examples: Ingestion of raw meat (including raw-hide treats and wildlife, through predation) Lack of prophylactic endo- and ectoparasiticide administration Lack of vaccination

food hygiene measures recommended for the handling of raw meat. That is not to say that dogs fed cooked diets do not develop campylobacteriosis or salmonellosis, do not shed food-poisoning associated bacteria, or do not carry AMR bacteria; it is just that the risk of this is lower.

5.5.2 Options for risk management

Risk management can be divided into easily manageable stages (Fig. 5.3).

The first step is to become *aware* that there is a risk, infectious disease is common, risk of infectious disease increases as population densities increase (multifactorial), and zoonotic infection will occur wherever humans and animals interact.

The next step is to *identify* the potential pathogens present within the animal population(s) under review. Other species present within the environment should be considered, as potential reservoirs or sentinels. The likelihood of disease importation should also be considered (function of frequency of travel and frequency of infection within the travelled). This can be through review of diseases or pathogens reported by others typically under similar circumstances for the same geographical location and same (or similar) species of animal, through screening of the population for the presence of pathogens (either directly or indirectly), and audit of recorded disease within the population. Review of diseases or pathogens reported by others can be useful in identifying risks for which control measures are already in place (e.g. widespread vaccination) resulting in low frequency of disease; this can also be used to identify non-endemic infections. Screening of the population is the costliest method of identifying pathogens present and is limited by the sensitivity and specificity of test modalities applied and numbers of tests performed. It is most likely to miss pathogens of low prevalence or where there is low test sensitivity. Audit of disease is reliant on an accurate database and gives only a historical view of disease prevalence; however, it is more likely to identify low-frequency incidents.

Identified risks are subsequently *assessed*, considering morbidity and mortality of the disease itself, the likelihood of transmission through various routes and the prevalence within the population (see Fig. 5.3). Diseases that are of high morbidity/mortality are prioritized, especially if they are of significant zoonotic potential or economic importance, as are those of high prevalence/transmission risk. Various methods to *control* the risks are evaluated. Selected controls are *implemented* and their efficacy is evaluated through *monitoring*.

One method of control is to screen animals for the presence of a communicable disease, with isolation of suspected or proven infected animals (to limit further transmission) for treatment or removal from the population (for example, rehoming to a household or population where infection is considered acceptable, or euthanasia where this is not possible). This is particularly applicable for infections where a subclinical state is common (e.g. FIV infection in cats; bTB in cattle). Alongside vaccination, screening for FeLV infection has

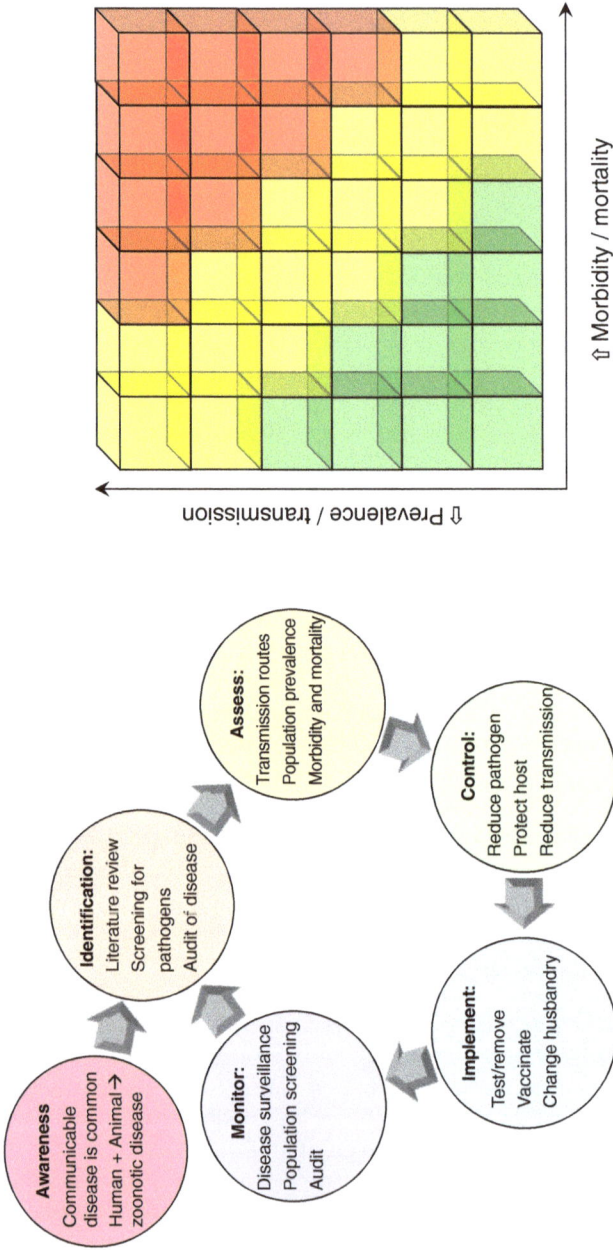

Fig. 5.3. Stages of risk management applied to communicable disease. Risk is often considered as a function of the morbidity/mortality and prevalence/rate of transmission.

been particularly successful in the reduction of FeLV-associated disease and infection prevalence in the pedigree cat population. Where pathogen prevalence is being actively managed within a specific population, animals are ideally screened before they enter, following potential exposure events, and, in some cases, periodically as part of regular surveillance, as suggested by the Human Animal Infections and Risk Surveillance group (HAIRS) (available at: https://www.gov.uk/government/collections/human-animal-infections-and-risk-surveillance-group-hairs, accessed June 2022).

5.5.3   Testing for communicable disease pathogens

The ideal screening test will be accurate (i.e. have both high sensitivity and high specificity), be simple to perform, produce rapid results, and be cost effective. Ideally, the presence of the organism is confirmed by direct visualization, culture, antigen detection (e.g. FeLV antigen screening in cats) or genetic material detection (e.g. PCR for pathogenic *Leptospira* spp.). Sometimes this is not possible (e.g. the organism is uncultivatable), practical (e.g. it takes months for the culture), or accurate. In these situations, exposure to an organism can be inferred by evaluating host response, either in the form of serum antibody testing (e.g. FIV antibody screening in cats) or assessment of cell-mediated immunity (e.g. tuberculin skin testing in cattle, or interferon gamma release assay in dogs and cats for mycobacteriosis). However, the host response is variable, and not always a useful marker for infection (i.e. a positive result may just indicate prior exposure or vaccine response and is reliant on there being a functional immune system). During acute infection, antibodies can be seen to appear (seroconversion), markedly increase in concentration ($\geq$ fourfold rising titre), or switch type from IgM to IgG (class switch). However, the timing of these events can vary between individuals and infectious agents, and comparison of results requires accurate quantitative measurements by the same technique. Where pathogen prevalence is high and chronic carrier state common, the significance of a single positive result becomes questionable. In such cases, qualitative tests are often used prior to more invasive, expensive, or time-consuming tests or are interpreted in conjunction with clinical signs.

The focus of most screening tests is sensitivity – to identify all infected animals. Ideally, positive results are then confirmed using more specific assays – to identify false-positive results, especially where the positive predictive value was low due to low prevalence or being clinically normal or the stakes are high (for example, a positive result would lead to their removal from the genetic pool or euthanasia). However, more specific assays may be limited by sensitivity (i.e. risk of false negative result) or practicality (e.g. require collection of post-mortem samples). Under these circumstances a cost–benefit analysis is made.

Boxes 5.1 and 5.2 give examples of testing for communicable diseases.

Box 5.1. Example of communicable disease: *Mycobacterium bovis* infection (bTB) in cattle.

bTB in cattle has significant economic and One Health impact and allows highlighting of the many complexities of communicable disease. Over 43,000 cattle were slaughtered in the UK in 2019 affecting >5% of herds in England and Wales. The subclinical phase of infection is long, and during this time cattle may be infectious. bTB can also infect other mammals, including wildlife, domestic pets and humans (Fig. 5.4).

Transmission occurs via inhalation or ingestion of infected material (respiratory tract excretions, urine, meat, or unpasteurized milk). Wildlife can act as a reservoir of infection and likely represent a significant source of infection to pets. Pets can be a source of infection to their owners as well as each other, including nosocomial transmission.

The tuberculin test is used to identify cattle with bTB, by evaluating host response to *M. bovis* proteins. Dependent upon the herd history, measurements are interpreted using either 'standard criteria' or 'severe criteria' with results considered negative, positive, or inconclusive. Interpretation using 'severe criteria' has increased sensitivity, offset by decreased specificity. Testing strategies and methods vary across species, further increasing complexity.

This is a high-stakes process: positive cattle are slaughtered, while inconclusive cattle are isolated then retested after 2 months (and slaughtered if positive or still inconclusive). Negative cattle are retested according to the farm's testing regimen. Regardless of interpretation criteria used, both false-positive and false-negative results will occur.

Alternative control methods (e.g. vaccination) have been debated, but their application is limited: (i) concurrent control of bTB in the sylvatic reservoir would be required alongside control in cattle; (ii) vaccination of cattle against bTB would require a change in legislation; (iii) vaccinated cattle cannot be differentiated from concurrently infected cattle; and (iv) currently available vaccines are only effective in 60–70% of cattle.

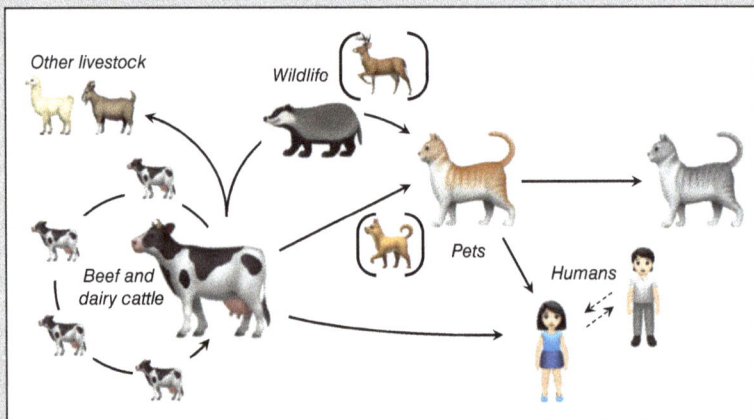

Fig. 5.4. Transmission routes of bTB.

Continued

Box 5.1. Continued.

The debate on how to best manage bTB remains controversial, with many different stakeholders involved, including vets, farmers, livestock handlers, consumers, wildlife guardians, pet owners and animals.

Box 5.2. Example of communicable disease: *Brucella canis* infection in dogs.

Brucellosis is a chronic systemic bacterial infection with a worldwide distribution. Although there is some degree of host preference, most *Brucella* spp. have the potential to cause life-changing severe disease in animals and people. *In vivo*, organisms are primarily intracellular, which results in immune system evasion and limits the effect of antimicrobials. However, *Brucella* spp. are capable of extracellular survival. Zoonotic infections follow unprotected handling of infected animals and material (e.g. abortion products), ingestion of contaminated dairy products, or following bacterial isolation in diagnostic laboratories.

Brucellosis in dogs is primarily caused by bacterium *Brucella canis*. The clinical signs most frequently relate to reproductive disorders (epididymo-orchitis; still-birth; abortion), discospondylitis (spinal pain; neurological deficits), or uveitis (painful, non-visual eye). Non-specific signs relating to a systemic inflammatory response (enlarged lymph nodes; painful joints; pyrexia) may also be seen. Subclinical infection is common and subtle signs of disease are easily missed (e.g. persistent or recurrent preputial or vulval discharge, and infertility), significantly contributing to the reservoir of disease. Until recently, it was rarely considered as a significant differential diagnosis in the UK. Bacterial shedding occurs within bodily fluids (e.g. preputial or vulval discharge; urine; milk) and can be persistent, with infection following ingestion of infected material, or via contamination of mucous membranes or wounds. Both vertical and horizontal (especially venereal) transmission occurs in dogs.

Prevalence of canine brucellosis in Western Europe is relatively low; however, recorded numbers of cases, including in the UK, are increasing due to a combination of increased travel and clinical awareness. Over the past decade there have been a small number of outbreaks associated with breeding kennels in Europe and North America.

The decision to test for brucellosis is based upon a combination of clinical signs, history of breeding, travel and possible exposure events. Currently, there is no legal framework to mandate testing for brucellosis prior to travel into the UK and recently exposed dogs may not have had sufficient time to seroconvert, necessitating repeat testing. In clinical cases, most screening serological tests offer good to excellent sensitivity, which if positive and combined with clinical suspicion of brucellosis will strongly support a diagnosis. However, in healthy dogs (where the suspicion of infection is low) the potential for serological false-positive results becomes an issue, while the sensitivity of definitive tests (i.e. PCR and culture) is poor.

Treatment of canine brucellosis is controversial. Euthanasia is commonly recommended on the grounds of: (i) ethical concern (painful clinical conditions; need to isolate infected dogs); (ii) antimicrobial stewardship (no proven curative

Continued

> **Box 5.2.** Continued.
>
> protocol; use of human antimicrobials; extended courses required); and (iii) public
> health (zoonotic risk). However, euthanasia is not legally enforceable, and owners
> might be resistant to euthanize a dog they consider to be healthy, especially if
> 'rescued' in the first place.

5.6   Influence of Healthcare on Communicable Disease

5.6.1   Overview

Preventive healthcare, when applied to communicable disease, typically takes
the form of vaccination and selective antimicrobial administration (e.g. regular
deworming). Good husbandry practices and hygiene are also important as preventive healthcare. Through these mechanisms communicable disease can
be reduced; however, they are not without limitation and unintended consequences that need to be considered.

Healthcare can also contribute to communicable disease. In bringing sick
individuals with communicable disease into the same environment as those
that are vulnerable either due to young age and immunological naivety or
immunocompromise, there is the risk of nosocomial transmission. Treatment
modalities (e.g. cytotoxic agents) may suppress the host immune response,
making individuals more vulnerable to infection. Antimicrobials may also
select for pathogens that are resistant to routine treatments and unbalance the
resident microbiota, providing a niche into which resistant organisms can col-
onize. There is also increasing concern that excreted antimicrobials, including
prophylactic ecto- and endoparasiticides, can contribute to environmental
contamination and selective pressure for antimicrobial resistance.

5.6.2   Vaccination

Vaccination has repeatedly been shown to be highly effective at reducing communicable disease. Vaccination is the administration of an antigenic product
to stimulate an adaptive immune response against a target pathogen. The level
of 'immunity' achieved is variable:

- **Sterilizing** (preferable) – where the individual is unable to become infected
  following exposure and does not develop clinical signs.
- **Non-sterilizing** – where infection, clinical signs and transmission are still
  possible, albeit with reduced likelihood and severity.

Herd immunity is where a sufficient level of immunity is present within
a population to minimize the risk of onward transmission. The percentage of
immune individuals within a population required to achieve herd immunity is

dependent upon the transmissibility of a pathogen, including its persistence within the environment, its presence in 'reservoir' species, as well as whether sterilizing immunity is possible following vaccination or initial exposure. Taken to an extreme, eradication of some pathogens becomes possible, while for others it is not possible to achieve herd immunity.

There are limitations to the use of vaccination, necessitating a cost–benefit analysis prior to application. There are inherent costs in the design, manufacture, transport, storage and administration of vaccines. Benefits include a reduction in morbidity and mortality in the animals vaccinated (for example, rabies vaccination of dogs reduces their risk) as well as a reduction in transmission to others (for example, rabies vaccination of dogs reduces the risk of rabies in children; vaccination of layer hens against salmonellosis reduces the risk of salmonellosis in humans). Use of some vaccines is subject to legal frameworks (for example, routine rabies vaccination in dogs is a legal require- ment in some countries and in others a requirement of travel across selected international borders) or are required to enable access to certain markets or facilities (for example, vaccination of dogs against *Bordetella bronchiseptica* prior to kennelling; vaccination of horses against equine influenza prior to competition). In contrast, use of vaccination against some infectious diseases is banned (see Box 5.1).

For both humans and veterinary species, guidelines exist detailing which vaccines should be administered and when (Day *et al.*, 2016). Some vaccines are considered as core (i.e. should be given to all regardless of circumstance) or non-core (i.e. should only be given to certain populations under certain conditions due to increased risk of exposure or morbidity/mortality). These guidelines often contain recommendations as to vaccination schedules, which aim to minimize the window of susceptibility and take account of maternally derived passive immunity, requirement for repeated challenge, and duration of immunity following vaccination. Maternal immunity can be enhanced by annual booster vaccination of the dam prior to breeding, and its interference in response to vaccination is not an indicator of poor husbandry. On an in- dividual basis, response to vaccination may be determined using serological tests for antibody levels and can be used to determine the requirement for an extended primary vaccination course or booster. However, such testing is not applicable to all vaccines, as cell-mediated immunity may be the predominant mechanism of protection.

It should be remembered that vaccination does not prevent disease in all cases, even where manufacturers' guidelines are followed. Vaccination failure may be seen due to both avoidable errors and idiosyncratic reasons.

5.6.3 Antimicrobial administration

A variety of antimicrobial agents are administered to individuals and more generally within a population to limit the impact and spread of communicable disease. In the absence of prior infection this is considered prophylactic. This includes ecto- and endoparasiticides (e.g. against fleas, biting flies, ticks and helminths). These parasites may themselves cause pathology, or result in the vector-borne transmission of pathogenic organisms (e.g. *B. burgdorferi* by ticks; *L. infantum* by *Phlebotomus* spp. sandflies). When formulating a treatment schedule the respective durations of action against the relevant parasites should be considered, to ensure sustained protection. The mechanism of action should also be considered; where pathogens are rapidly transmitted during haematophagous arthropod activity the agent selected should be repellent. The activity of surface agents that act on contact might be impacted by washing of the coat, while haematophagous activity itself could cause pathology (e.g. pruritus).

As with antibacterials, with regular and sustained use of prophylactic parasiticides there is concern regarding both resistance and environmental contamination. There has been a trend towards reactive use rather than prophylactic use, with performance of faecal analysis (e.g. egg counts) to assess for the presence of infestation prior to treatment. Unfortunately, for some parasitic diseases (e.g. angiostrongylosis in dogs) clinical signs can precede patent (i.e. detectable) infection.

Various veterinary guidelines, such as BSAVA's PROTECT-ME (Allerton, 2018) and the International Society for Companion Animal Infectious Diseases (ISCAID) guidelines (Weese *et al.*, 2019), have been produced to promote antimicrobial stewardship and minimize the impact of antimicrobial resistance on human and veterinary populations. These guidelines promote use of antimicrobials solely for the treatment of specific infections (i.e. not for prophylaxis or growth promotion), making decisions based on antimicrobial resistance patterns, and selection of appropriate doses and duration of usage. There is increasing concern in the medical and geopolitical arena regarding the contribution of antimicrobial use in animals to antimicrobial resistance, particularly where these antimicrobials are used prophylactically, indiscriminately, or for growth promotion. In some European countries, certain classes of antimicrobials (e.g. fluoroquinolones) have been banned for use in veterinary species, while in other countries rules restrict their use to specific circumstances. These efforts have reduced antimicrobial usage per capita and levels of antimicrobial resistance; however, it does limit treatment options and has the potential to negatively impact on an individual animal's quality of life. Other countries have used a softer approach, banning the use of antimicrobials for growth promotion, but not nationally limiting the use of specific antimicrobials for treatment purposes. Implementation of stricter legal restrictions to veterinary prescribing could be considered justified if there is indiscriminate use of antimicrobials. Therefore, it is important that the veterinary profession applies a One Health approach and visibly promotes antimicrobial stewardship, including in the care of companion animals. For most of the general public, companion animal care provides their most visible examples of responsible veterinary antimicrobial usage.

Education of others is an important part of antimicrobial stewardship. This may take the form of raising awareness of antimicrobial resistance: how it develops, why it is a growing concern, and how it can be limited (for example: not using antimicrobials in every animal; not using them prophylactically; using the appropriate dose and course for the infection present). Raising awareness can be through waiting-room posters, leaflets, or the practice website. It can also include signposting the practice's antimicrobial usage policy to owners requesting medication or while discharging patients on antimicrobial medication. In human primary care settings (which perhaps better translates to veterinary small animal first-opinion practice), it has been shown that the use of 'storytelling' and visual personal commitment (such as a poster with your photo and commitment to responsible antimicrobial use) is one of the simplest and most effective measures that can be taken. Becoming a practice antimicrobial champion and promoting antimicrobial stewardship can be a role undertaken by veterinary nurses or animal care assistants. For greater impact, in-practice campaigns can coincide with other local One Health initiatives (e.g. in human pharmacies or NHS GP surgeries) or with the World Health Organization's World Antimicrobial Awareness Week (18–24 November) (available at https://www.who.int/campaigns/world-antimicrobial-awareness-week, accessed June, 2022) and the European Centre for Disease Prevention and Control's annual European Antibiotic Awareness Day (18 November).

5.6.4 Environmental factors

Good husbandry plays an important part in the management of communicable diseases. Animals should be kept in conditions that are well maintained, easy to clean and disinfect, with good ventilation and rapid waste removal. However, increased stocking density is often necessary to maximize usage of limited space. While stocking density is a term more typically applied to intensive farming, the same principles and problems apply to breeding or boarding catteries and kennels (including 'puppy farms'), animal shelters, veterinary practices and hoarders. Increasing stocking density increases the risk of communicable disease through several mechanisms. More animals mean more waste, including carbon dioxide, faeces and urine. Uncontrolled accumulation of waste products contributes to increased stress and increased environmental contamination. Risk of transmission increases as the environment becomes more contaminated, direct contact between animals increases and greater numbers share the same airspace. Increased stress increases risk of disease following exposure and increased pathogen shedding when infected. To mitigate the impact of increased stocking density, increased levels of resources per unit area are required to remove waste and limit pathogens transmission; however, resources increase overheads.

Within individual establishments, groups of animals at different life stages should be housed separately in stable groups with limited mixing. Older animals can represent sources of infection to naïve younger animals. Reduced exposure to alternative sources of infection (e.g. wildlife; visiting cats and dogs) and use of quarantine facilities for incoming animals can also reduce the risk of infectious disease within a household.

Within a veterinary hospital, boarding kennel or cattery, contact between animals from different households should be limited, especially for cats where subclinical carriage of respiratory viruses is common. This can be achieved by use of separate air spaces and sneeze barriers. Where potentially infectious cases are seen, dedicated facilities should be used, with additional time for thorough cleaning factored into the use of shared amenities.

Access points for shared resources (e.g. food, water, waste removal) can be sites of contamination. When planning the construction or refurbishment of a facility anticipated to hold a large number of animals in close proximity to each other, close attention should be paid to the central positioning of resources, limiting of transmission routes between the individual units within which an animal will be placed, ensuring that the units (including outdoor runs) can be easily and individually cleaned and disinfected appropriately, and including facilities to isolate or barrier-nurse animals separately. At the opposite end of the spectrum, where there has been an outbreak of disease, an on-site assessment of the facilities and observation of daily routine are often required to identify all potential routes of transmission and sources of infection.

5.7 Reporting of Communicable Diseases

Finally, we need to recognize that some communicable diseases are legally reportable. The list of reportable diseases will vary from country to country, within years, and between species. The purpose of this reporting is multifactorial: it allows the monitoring of impact of control measures, highlights which diseases are increasing in prevalence, and ensures that appropriate measures are taken to limit onward spread of diseases with often significant human or economic impact. It is the responsibility of the veterinary professionals (either in practice or in laboratory settings) to report diagnosis of these diseases to the relevant public health authorities.

5.8 Summary

Communicable disease is a fascinating aspect of One Health. Through its lens we can look at human–animal interactions, pathology, immunology, pharmacology, diagnostic techniques, economics, legislation and more. It is a huge, dynamic, constantly shifting topic, whose surface can barely be scratched; therefore, regular review of the literature is essential to update the evidence base upon which we make our decisions.

5.9 Questions for Further Discussion

1. Canine infectious respiratory disease complex (CIRDC) or 'kennel cough' is a common empirical diagnosis for acute-onset cough in first-opinion small animal practice. How would you explain to a client why one of their dogs could have been diagnosed with 'kennel cough' despite having received its vaccine 'booster' 6 months earlier and having not recently been in kennels?

2. Feline calicivirus virulent systemic disease is a rare manifestation of infection with a common respiratory tract infectious agent. Outbreaks are associated with a very high mortality rate and often include pets owned by veterinary staff members. Given how this infectious agent is spread, consider how you would manage an outbreak of feline calicivirus virulent systemic disease in the practice you work at or most recently visited.

3. There is increasing interest regarding faecal matter transplantation as a treatment of intestinal disease in a variety of species. Consider the potential infectious disease risks associated with such a practice and how these risks could be mitigated against. What would be your 'ideal donor' animal?

5.10 Case Study: Treacle the French bulldog

5.10.1 Case description

Treacle (name changed), a 12-week-old male entire French bulldog, was presented with a recent history of lethargy and inappetence, and haemorrhagic diarrhoea. He had no history of travel, had been in the owner's possession for 2 weeks, and had received his first dose of a live multivalent vaccine (containing canine distemper virus, canine parvovirus, canine adenovirus type 2, canine parainfluenza virus) combined with an inactivated *Leptospira* vaccine 10 days earlier. He was fed a commercial raw diet. He had access to a private garden but had not been walked off the property. Another dog in the household was clinically well.

On physical examination, Treacle was dehydrated and pyrexic (39.7°C).

5.10.2 Differential diagnoses

Infectious causes of lethargy, inappetence and diarrhoea considered included viral (e.g. canine parvovirus; canine distemper), bacterial (e.g. salmonellosis; campylobacteriosis) and parasitic (e.g. cryptosporidiosis; hook worms; *Giardia* spp.), possibly with systemic compromise (e.g. sepsis). Fungal, oomycete and algal infections were considered extremely unlikely. Non-infectious differential diagnoses also considered included dietary indiscretion, dietary change, systemic disease (e.g. portosystemic shunt and hepatic encephalopathy; hypoadrenocorticism) and

Continued

Case Study Continued.

structural intestinal disease (e.g. foreign body; intussusception; cancer). Co-morbidities are common in young dogs, so an open mind was kept.

Canine parvovirus was a significant differential as both a common cause of gastrointestinal disease in incompletely vaccinated puppies and due to its potential for nosocomial spread. Viral particles can survive in the environment for a long time, while veterinary staff and fomites can be vectors. While most dogs with parvovirosis present with vomiting and haemorrhagic diarrhoea, some present peracutely (i.e. before the onset of these signs) or with more subtle signs. Salmonellosis and campylobacteriosis were also significant differentials, due to Treacle's young age and raw diet. Faecal shedding of *Salmonella* spp. or *Campylobacter* spp. organisms can also cause both nosocomial and zoonotic transmission.

5.10.3 Investigation

Blood analysis (haematology and serum biochemistry) was performed, and faeces were submitted for direct visualization of parasites, selective culture of bacteria, detection of pathogen antigens (viral and parasitic), and PCR (viral, bacterial, and parasitic). Some tests were performed at point-of-care (e.g. lateral flow antigen test for canine parvovirus), with the advantage of rapidly identifying the presence of important infectious agents. Abdominal ultrasound was performed to assess for structural disease.

Haematology revealed a pancytopenia, comprising a moderate non-regenerative anaemia, thrombocytopenia and mild neutropenia with left shift and marked toxic change. Possibilities for the pancytopenia included bone marrow injury, immune-mediated destruction and ongoing losses. The left-shift neutropenia with toxic change was of greatest cause of concern as it suggested acute overwhelming inflammation. Cytopenias are commonly seen with parvovirosis through a combination of bone marrow injury, gastrointestinal haemorrhage and sepsis. Salmonellosis, campylobacteriosis and other severe systemic infections can also result in similar changes. Serum biochemistry also revealed evidence of an acute-phase inflammatory response or gastrointestinal losses, with a marked hypoalbuminaemia.

Abdominal ultrasound revealed prominent mesenteric lymph nodes and mild, non-specific changes to the small intestinal wall – common changes in young dogs.

In-house faecal analysis was weakly positive for canine parvovirus by antigen ELISA. Externally submitted pooled faecal samples were positive for canine parvovirus by PCR, *Giardia* spp. by antigen ELISA and direct visualization, *Cryptosporidium* spp. antigen by enzyme immunoassay, and *Salmonella enterica* serotype Dublin by culture. Note: *Salmonella* spp. infection in dogs is now reportable by the veterinary laboratories that culture it in the UK.

Due to persistent pyrexia and haematological changes, blood culture was also performed. This revealed *Salmonella* spp. septicaemia.

Continued

Case Study Continued.

5.10.4 Minimizing the potential risk of disease transmission

Treacle was barrier-nursed pending results (i.e. as if he was shedding parvovirus or *Salmonella* spp.). Movement around the practice was minimized and Treacle was isolated from others in a demarcated area with dedicated equipment (e.g. stethoscope, thermometer, leash) and outdoor areas to defecate and urinate. Dirty bedding was either disposed of or placed in vinegar bags and washed appropriately. Veterinary staff wore impermeable gowns, gloves and overshoes (or dedicated boots) to prevent contamination of their uniform. To treat the environment, after thorough cleaning, disinfectants active against parvovirus (including diluted bleach or Virkon) were used according to manufacturers' recommendations. Note: real grass can be difficult or impossible to disinfect adequately, while artificial grass can trap faecal particulate matter within its structure.

Following handling of Treacle and prior to touching the face or clinical records, hands were thoroughly washed with soap and water. Eating and drinking are routinely avoided in clinical areas.

5.10.5 Treatment, diagnosis and outcome

Treacle was administered fluid therapy and anti-nausea medication pending results. The diarrhoea resolved rapidly during hospitalization. The pyrexia resolved following antimicrobial administration and he went on to make a full recovery.

Treacle was ultimately diagnosed with salmonellosis, which had resulted in septicaemia. This was the likely cause of the persistent pyrexia, gastrointestinal signs and blood analysis changes. Not every dog with enteric *Salmonella* spp. carriage requires treatment (for example, those shedding *Salmonella* spp. in faeces with mild to no associated clinical signs); however, as Treacle had septicaemia, he was managed with antimicrobials supported by sensitivity results. His raw diet was considered a significant risk factor and he was transitioned to a commercial cooked diet. Concurrent parvovirosis could not be ruled out, but it was not considered a significant component of the clinical signs present. Severe haemorrhagic diarrhoea with cardiovascular collapse characterizes fulminant parvovirosis, but this was not seen. The positive parvovirus ELISA and PCR results could indicate: (i) a 'false-positive' result due to recent vaccination; or (ii) that Treacle was infected with a field-strain of canine parvovirus but had partial immunity. In dogs, faecal shedding of live virus following vaccination occurs at levels that should be detectable by antigen tests, while false-positive antigen results have been documented in cats following equivalent vaccination with live-attenuated feline panleukopenia virus. Treacle also had giardiasis and cryptosporidiosis. The significance of these two latter pathogens was unknown, particularly as some *Giardia* spp. and *Cryptosporidium* spp. species that infect dogs are potentially zoonotic, but not all. No specific treatment was given for the giardiasis and cryptosporidiosis, as these can be self-limiting and clinical signs had resolved.

References

Allerton, F. (2018) PROTECT-ME. Rationalizing antibacterials. *BSAVA Companion* 2018(11), 8–9.

Day, M.J., Horzinek, M.C., Schultz, R.D. and Squires, R.A. (2016) WSAVA Guidelines for the vaccination of dogs and cats. *Journal of Small Animal Practice* 57, 4–8. E1–E45.

Weese, J.S., Blondeau, J., Boothe, D., Guardabassi, L.G., Gumley, N. *et al.* (2019) International Society for Companion Animal Infectious Diseases (ISCAID) guidelines for the diagnosis and management of bacterial urinary tract infections in dogs and cats. *Veterinary Journal* 247, 8–25.

Public Health

6

Helen Ballantyne[1]*
[1]*NHS, Cambridge, UK*

Key Points

- What is public health?
- The framework for public health
- The relevance of public health to veterinary nursing
- Facilitating public health projects

6.1 What is Public Health?

Public health is perhaps one of the most relevant aspects of One Health for veterinary nurses (VNs). Engaging with public health is one of the simplest and arguably one of the most effective ways of supporting One Health in a practical and useful way. Many of the most well-known One Health projects have a public health theme: consider the collaborative work going on to deal with antibiotic resistance, the hand-washing posters that are displayed in both medical and veterinary hospitals as well as more specialist projects such as work on preventing dog bites in the community. It might be argued that public health is the very essence of One Health.

Despite this, it is probably also one of the most misunderstood elements of One Health. Within the veterinary profession, the phrase 'public health' often conjures up intimidating thoughts of massive global campaigns, eradication of disease, food safety and herd health, all of which may feel irrelevant and distant to most veterinary nurses, particularly when the majority of the veterinary nursing profession works in companion animal practice. The idea that veterinary public health is a discipline exclusively for veterinary surgeons is wrong but may be inadvertently reinforced by a lack of understanding of the basic concepts of public health medicine. Such misconceptions may result in

*Email: helen_ballantyne@yahoo.com

© CAB International 2023. *One Health for Veterinary Nurses and Technicians*
(eds R. Jones and A. Jeffery)
DOI: 10.1079/9781789249477.0006

missed opportunities to work within a One Health scope with potential benefits for all patients, their carers and the professionals involved.

This chapter offers a clear definition of public health and explains how and why it is more relevant to veterinary nursing than ever before. It explains why veterinary nurses are ideally placed to support public health and outlines the wide range of benefits that working within the public health discipline may offer to animals, people and professionals.

Before considering the concept of public health, there must be a clear understanding of the concept of health. While many definitions of health are offered, and readers can search and select the one that appeals, the critical point is that there has been a shift in the paradigm of health, which has been reflected in the role of the healthcare provider.

Early definitions of health centred on the absence of any flaw in a body, as a set of physiological systems, be that physical or mental flaws. Healthcare professionals were tasked with eliminating any flaws that might appear to blot the concept of 'health'.

More recently, as medicine and science have progressed offering a vast array of treatment options that are evolving daily, health as a concept has shifted to the idea that the physiological systems that make up a life form, be that human or animal, will be challenged and that the ability to manage those challenges make up the concept of health. As such, many healthcare professionals have seen their role adapt from being acute problem solvers to longer-term care givers and educators facilitating a patient's self-management. This shift in paradigm applies equally to human-centred nurses and veterinary nurses.

The overarching feature of health is that it is a highly subjective concept. While it might be measured objectively through scoring of vital signs, weight, height, blood pressure, etc., one person's feeling healthy might well be another's unhealthy. Acknowledgement of this variability is a core component of nursing and may be the key difference between a medical and nursing approach. As an easy example, despite the potential for an identical diagnosis, health and recovery for a premier league footballer will look quite different to the 44-year-old office worker who likes to play five-aside with his mates on a Thursday night. The owner of a prize-winning thoroughbred will be looking for a different version of health for their animal than the owner of an elderly cob who hacks out every other Sunday.

The medical model of care provides a diagnosis and associated treatment plan; it is objective and transactional. A nursing approach must look wider in a holistic manner. It is up to nurses to know and understand the detail that surrounds the patient, the factors that are contributing to ill health and the resources available to combat it. Doctors and vets may observe a set of blood tests and diagnose diabetes mellitus; a nurse has a duty to know and understand so much more about that patient and their owner. They need to consider and incorporate the patient's and owner's lifestyles, their support networks, their culture and their values, to ensure that care plans are unique and relevant to that patient.

Approaching a patient within the One Health context supports holistic nursing. It offers the opportunity to optimize how nurses may support their patients back to their version of health. It might be as simple as a human-centred nurse enquiring if the family has a dog, to start a conversation about the benefits of exercise for a newly diabetic patient, or as basic as a veterinary nurse taking the time to learn more about the owner of the animal they are treating to understand their attitudes to health. If an owner is obese and admits to living off take-away food which they share with their dog, there is an immediate and significant barrier to any intervention a veterinary nurse may want to put in place to facilitate weight loss for that dog.

The World Health Organization defines Public Health as '*the art and science of preventing disease, prolonging life, and promoting health through the organised efforts of society*' (Acheson, 1988; WHO, 1999). Veterinary nurses spend their working life trying to prevent disease and promote health, so hopefully this definition breaks down some of the misconceptions that public health is abstract, irrelevant or reserved for veterinary surgeons. Furthermore, if the word 'society' is taken in its basic form, it is a group of people. Society in this context is not just the broad term for an entire population, it can also mean a local focused society, society in a particular town or city or a group of people within a veterinary hospital.

All work within a public health context is characterized by being population focused, responsive to change, collaborative, scientific and holistic. Nursing shares these characteristics, meaning that VNs are ideally placed to instigate and develop public health and One Health projects to the benefit of their workplace, their community and their own professional development.

Veterinary public health has its own definition from the WHO, written in collaboration with the Food and Agriculture Organization of the United Nations (FAO), which says: '*the sum of all contributions to the physical, mental, and social wellbeing of humans through an understanding and application of veterinary science*' (WHO, 1999). A list of examples of direct responsibilities of veterinary public health is provided in Box 6.1. The use of the term 'veterinary science' is relevant to nurses considering their role in public health, for it broadens the scope and invites anyone who is willing to ensure that they are working in an informed and evidence-based manner to participate. There are many opportunities for veterinary nurses to support and promote public health.

It is highly likely that many veterinary nurses reading this chapter will already be involved in public health projects, but that due to the misconception

---

Box 6.1. Direct responsibilities of veterinary public health.

- Promotion of animal health in relation to the food chain and food security
- Surveillance of disease, particularly in relation to zoonosis
- Consideration of the environmental impact of veterinary medicine
- Animal trade and movement
- Promotion and consideration of the human–animal bond

of the term public health, the work they have been doing has never been considered as public health.

For example, veterinary nurses are with vets on the frontline of the detection, testing and surveillance of zoonotic conditions. Once a formal diagnosis is in place, it is often the veterinary nursing team who are responsible for the subsequent isolation, quarantine and infection control measures required to care for such an animal. Such tasks are critical to prevent infection transmission and the associated skill base required is diverse and complex.

Many veterinary nurses are already playing a role in public health through their professional interest in protecting the environment, which is an equal element of the One Health triad. Consideration of the impact of veterinary work on the environment can be considered a public health duty. At the time of writing, a debate regarding the environmental impact of some parasitic treatments has begun. Veterinary hospitals are striving to reduce their use of single-use plastic and to support greener alternatives. Veterinary nurses are well placed to take on leadership roles in this area (for further information see Chapter 7, Environmental Sustainability in Veterinary Practice).

Finally, the strength and mutual benefit of the human–animal bond is well documented to benefit the health of the pet owners, and, as such, does not every interaction with a companion animal in veterinary practice have the aim of enriching the life of both animal and client? To support the health and wellbeing of both? It is difficult to support the healthcare needs of an animal without taking the owner's needs into account (see Chapter 3, The Human–Animal Bond).

6.1.1   Prevent, Promote and Pursue – public health for veterinary nurses in a One Health context

Using the definition of public health from WHO, a framework of public health emerges that may be used within the One Health context: Prevent, Promote and Pursue – the prevention of disease, the promotion of health and the pursuit of quality of life. Each element covers a key part of public health, with practical applications listed in Table 6.1.

Prevention is the principle of reducing the incidence and the impact of disease. This will incorporate immunization and support of public health campaigns such as hand washing, alongside the support of widespread surveillance and monitoring of disease profiles. A local example may be intervening when dog fouling is a problem in a particular area, through the provision of poo bags and relevant education.

Promotion of health is the second part of the framework. Health promotion in One Health is not about veterinary nurses advising the owners of animals about their health and wellbeing, or human-centred nurses advising about animals; it is about staying within a professional scope of practice and thinking holistically. A truly holistic approach to any patient care will be a

Table 6.1. Public health framework in practice.

Prevent ill health	**Promote** health	**Pursue** quality of life
Vaccination programmes (Prevention of disease and positive healthcare modelling for medicine)	Use of the Five Welfare Needs for animals: diet, environment, health, companionship and behaviour	Acknowledgement of the human–animal bond (Support to a bereaved owner, participation in outreach clinic for the pets of homeless community)
Participation in reporting and surveillance of new and emerging disease patterns, keeping up to date with legislation and guidance for animals moving internationally (Prevention of new and emerging disease, ability to highlight and take measures if new diseases emerge)	Education and promotion of participation in vaccination programmes (Indirect support of government-supported vaccination regimens)	Working with owners to support the care of patients with chronic conditions (Reassurance allows those struggling with immunosuppression to spend time with their pets without feeling fearful; benefit to both animals and patient)
Health checks	Research and acknowledgement and incorporation of local social determinants of health into veterinary team business plan	
Administration of barrier nursing care to a dog with suspect infectious disease	Obesity	
Infection control measures established for a zoonotic disease	Passive smoking	
Support for global/local healthcare campaigns (e.g. hand washing)		
Pre-purchase education for a family considering buying a puppy		

One Health approach, as it is about understanding that education about an animal's health and wellbeing may well have a positive impact on an owner's health and wellbeing and vice versa.

Here the obvious example is smoking cessation. Those owners who are educated about the dangers of second-hand smoke to their pets may take steps towards reducing or even stopping smoking. Smoking-related healthcare problems account for a massive proportion of healthcare resource and while the numbers of people who smoke are declining, the public health implications of those who remain addicted to the habit are real (see Chapter 4, Non-Communicable Diseases and Other Shared Health Risks). If VNs can contribute towards a reduction in those problems, this is public health in action, albeit as a secondary benefit to the primary aim of improving the health of an animal.

Health promotion within human-centred nursing has been studied extensively, as poor lifestyle choices contribute to increasing numbers of people with preventable diseases. Using health psychology and tried-and-tested health promotion techniques, patients may be supported to make healthier choices around diet, exercise and alcohol intake, for example. This is all valuable experience and knowledge which might be used and applied by veterinary nurses working with owners of animals suffering from the same sort of lifestyle-associated problems, obesity in animals being the most common example.

The final part of the framework is an adaptation of the phrase 'prolong life' as used by the WHO definition of public health. In the One Health context, this is too simplistic a phrase as it does not allow for the veterinary sector, where euthanasia may be a valid treatment option. While human medicine may have individual cases of patients who decline specific treatments and, if treatment is deemed futile for some serious health conditions, then treatment may be withdrawn by the medical team, the basic overriding principle in human healthcare is to prolong life at all costs. This is not the approach in veterinary medicine.

As with the concept of health, quality of life is highly subjective. Within human-centred nursing, staff are encouraged to work in a 'patient-centred' approach to ensure that any decisions are made with the patient's involvement. The aim is to ensure that elements of a patient's life that might be deemed critical to their quality of life are incorporated into care plans.

The all-important human–animal bond sits within this part of the framework, alongside consideration of the care of animals with long-term conditions. It might be argued that this is one of the areas where collaborative practice between healthcare professionals has the most potential to support the mutual health and wellbeing of both animals and humans through the sharing of resources, education and learning.

The development of guidelines for animals in healthcare settings as provided by the Royal College of Nursing (RCN, 2019) is an excellent example of collaborative practice that hopes to increase the number of volunteers willing to visit patients in hospitals with their dogs. Such visits have the potential to improve the quality of life for patients in hospitals, provide fulfilment for the owners of the dogs and the dogs themselves, as well as brightening the day of the medical staff on shift when the therapy dogs visit.

6.2 Why is Public Health Relevant to Veterinary Nursing?

Public health is becoming more relevant to human-centred nursing for three main reasons. Firstly, there is an ongoing dynamic shift in healthcare priority from managing acute health needs to chronic care for people with long-term conditions. This shift in paradigm calls for a collective approach that incorporates health promotion, education and long-term care planning.

Secondly, more people are being cared for in the community. An ageing population with chronic co-morbidities require ongoing support and care that can be managed in their own home. A combination of patient choice, patient safety and recognition of the need to preserve hospital beds means patients with increasingly complex needs are being cared for by ambulatory nurses in the community.

Finally, the digital age has enabled vast amounts of health-related data to be collected and analysed. Subsequently there is a greater ability to predict health problems before they occur. It is recognized that factors such as housing and the environment, income, level of education, employment conditions, known as social determinants of health, may impact more on people's health needs than their own lifestyle choices or local healthcare provision. In the author's hometown for example, there is an overrepresentation of orthopaedic interventions, fractured bones, hips, legs, wrists. When this is considered with the knowledge that the town's biggest employer is the horse-racing industry, the data is logical. Commissioning groups who have a duty to assess such needs might well decide that the town in question requires higher levels of rehabilitation care and offer more funding for physiotherapy.

With this knowledge comes a duty of care to act: now that healthcare problems might be predictable in certain areas of the country with certain demographic groups, a public health strategy can and should be designed to prevent the problem.

The increased relevance of public health is pertinent to veterinary medicine too. Just like people, animals are living longer, with increasingly complex healthcare needs. The general public has an increasing level of health literacy and will look to the veterinary care of their animals to be comparable to that which they receive. Veterinary professionals have a duty to think broadly about the preventive healthcare approach and educate and support owners to prevent disease and optimize their pet's health.

An increase in the number of people receiving increasingly complex care for long-term conditions in the community may also have a direct impact on veterinary professionals and trigger a need to have a broader understanding of issues impacting their clients. Owners who are receiving care for long-term conditions are much more likely to require extra support to care for their animals. Veterinary interventions cannot be instructions issued in isolation; the owner's needs must also be considered. They must be able to follow through with a care plan physically and cognitively.

Finally, it might be argued that the social determinants of health are as relevant to veterinary practice as they are to a local doctor's surgery. Just as a local GP will analyse local social determinants of health to offer relevant services, so a veterinary practice that knows and understands some of the health issues that might be affecting people within a local community may offer an insight and an opportunity to support people and their pets. There are three main reasons why social determinants of health are relevant to veterinary practice: (i) the potential for improving healthcare outcomes; (ii) the opportunity for collaboration; and (iii) improvement of business planning and associated increased income stream.

Firstly, learning about the local social determinants of health is knowledge that may support therapeutic relationships and potentially improve veterinary healthcare outcomes. When caring for a patient with a long-term condition, for example, the development of a therapeutic relationship – one that is mutually respectful and engaged between veterinary nurse and owner – is essential to support whatever intervention is required to promote the health of the animal in question. Knowing and comprehending some of the issues relevant to the local community can support that therapeutic relationship, as care plans can be aligned accordingly and owners are more likely to engage with professionals who are empathetic to their own needs. So, if a veterinary practice is located close to a large city hospital, one of the most relevant social determinants of health might be the fact that many people may work at the hospital and consequently work shifts. Having this knowledge in the back of the mind will allow the nursing team to ensure that the care plans put in place are workable. A cat cannot receive medication three times a day if its owner is working 12½ h shifts.

Secondly, understanding the health needs of a community can support collaboration with human-centred or environmental agencies to potentially improve the health of both animals and people. Obesity is a common One Health theme with animals and people suffering from co-morbidities induced by being overweight; it is not uncommon for obese people to have obese pets. A collaborative approach, perhaps in a client evening format between veterinary and medical team, offers a broader viewpoint which may provide a novel approach to an old problem and encourage people to take action for themselves and their animals (see Chapter 4, Non-Communicable Diseases and Other Shared Health Risks).

Thirdly and finally, the incorporation of social determinants of health into a business plan or strategic modelling can potentially improve business income streams. Knowing the needs of a community may encourage closer client bonding, so that footfall through the practice increases, with associated increase in spending. Equally, knowing the needs and providing a relevant service is the age-old formula for making profit. For example, if a practice is situated in an area associated with high levels of poverty, a pet's health and wellbeing may be low down the list of priorities; offering payment plans might encourage people to engage more with the practice, to the benefit of their pet and their practice.

Researching and educating the practice team on local determinants of health may be considered an excellent opportunity for a veterinary nurse seeking a useful and relevant One Health project that allows them to develop professionally and support their local community.

The benefits of working within the public health context for the veterinary team are broad and may be categorized into professional, business and healthcare benefits (Table 6.2).

6.2.1   Healthcare outcomes

Awareness of the social determinants of health have the potential to optimize veterinary healthcare outcomes, as robust therapeutic relationships may be established between owners and nurses. Furthermore, knowing the needs of a community enables the veterinary team to meet those needs.

6.2.2   Professional benefits

A One Health approach which incorporates public health has the potential to offer professional development and fulfilment as well as the opportunity to specialize and pursue relevant further knowledge and education in a particular subject. A nurse who notices that many of their patients are coming into contact with second-hand smoke may develop an interest in trying to educate owners

Table 6.2. The benefits of working in public health.

Healthcare outcomes	Professional	Business
Improved therapeutic relationships	Professional development	Increased client engagement
Improved healthcare outcomes	CPD opportunities	Media interest, marketing/advertising
Meeting the needs of the local community	Opportunity to develop specialized knowledge	Improved confidence in discussing difficult topics with clients, including debt/finances
	Improved health and wellbeing	
	Reduction in work-based stress and anxiety	

about the dangers to their pets. There might be the opportunity to collaborate with a local GP practice, obtain some smoking cessation literature for the veterinary reception area, participate in accredited continued professional development (CPD) on behaviour change – all while working within their own scope of practice and promoting the health and wellbeing of the animal. Equally a veterinary nurse based in an area with a high elderly population might want to consider how the veterinary team might support pet owners with dementia; again, broadening their learning, perhaps completing online CPD borrowed from the medical profession, collaborating with agencies that specialize in dementia care.

Both are excellent examples of One Health projects that have the potential to benefit the animal, the owner and the professional by improving the health of the animal, the support to the owner and offering professional development and fulfilment to the nurse.

Engaging with public health can also help nursing staff cope with some of the more complex issues that may present in practice, potentially preventing them feeling stressed or anxious about a particular situation. The classic example in this case would be a nurse who feels concerned about a bereaved owner going home to an empty house with little support. If a veterinary team is already engaged with public health, they will be better placed to offer support, perhaps link the client with relevant local support services. Having the confidence and the resource to be able to do this can prevent team members feeling powerless and anxious about their clients – feelings which, if left unaddressed, could contribute to serious mental health problems.

Finally, a veterinary practice that is engaged with public health will be more informed about common contemporary healthcare issues. As such, staff may themselves seek support from their own healthcare providers if they recognize some of those issues in themselves. Again, obesity is an accessible and relevant example: bringing up the issue within the public health context may encourage members of the team to seek out their own solutions, such as exercising with colleagues, planned weekend team dog walks or support to attend slimming groups.

6.2.3   Business benefits

A veterinary team that understands the healthcare issues that its clients are facing will be better placed to support them as they in turn care for their animals. As such, it might be suggested that client engagement may be improved when there is a public health focus. Additionally, a focus on local healthcare through a One Health approach is also a way of working that is likely to be appealing to local media outlets, potentially providing free marketing and publicity.

Finally, a veterinary team that is engaged in public health will be potentially dealing with some sensitive issues, honing their communication skills and using recognized health promotion models. Such frameworks provide principles of communication that might be applied to other potentially sensitive issues in veterinary practice, including finances. Improved confidence discussing difficult topics may result in staff being more willing and able to tackle them, potentially improving the debt control within the practice as discussions are held in a full and frank manner instead of it being ignored.

6.3 What Can Veterinary Nurses Do?

6.3.1 Scope of practice

As has been demonstrated in this chapter, public health is a hugely broad and diverse topic. It would be very easy for VNs to believe that it does not concern them and that they simply need to concentrate on the patient, the animal presented to them, and ignore any overt issues with the owner. Furthermore, some might cite the Royal College of Veterinary Surgeons (RCVS) Code of Conduct, which mandates '*Veterinary nurses must keep within their own area of competence and refer cases responsibly*' as a reason not to engage with public health. This would be wrong.

Engaging with public health is not about working outside the veterinary nursing scope of practice; it is not asking veterinary nurses to work as human-centred nurses or vice versa. It is about taking the time to consider the bigger picture and think about how collaboration and shared knowledge may support better health outcomes for both animal and human.

Returning to the RCVS Code of Conduct (RCVS, 2014), section 2.1 says: '*Veterinary nurses must provide veterinary nursing care that is appropriate and adequate.*' It may be argued that this is impossible to do without considering the One Health and/or public health element of a client and their animal.

Prescribing care that cannot be implemented by the client due to either individual health problems or broader public health determinants like poverty will mean that the care given is neither appropriate nor adequate.

6.3.2 Sharing resources

Given the relevance and importance of public health to human-centred nursing, it should not come as a surprise to learn that there is a vast array of data and evidence to support several critical public health models, frameworks and techniques for nurses. Two in particular, 'Making every contact count' and 'Motivational interviewing', may be easily transferred and applied to veterinary nursing with the potential to assist direct veterinary nursing practice, or facilitate a direct step into public health within the context of veterinary nursing.

6.3.3 Making every contact count

This technique originated in 2008 with the aim of bringing public health into everyday healthcare practice. It is a mind-set used in human-centred nursing that supports professionals staying within their scope of practice, while encouraging them to consider every interaction with a patient as an opportunity to have a positive impact on their health and wellbeing. It is easier to explain with an example. Consider the work of a human-centred specialist allergy nurse. Their role is highly specific to their patient group, who require specialist knowledge and clinical skills. Yet, if a patient they are working with admits that they have stopped taking their prescribed blood pressure medication because they think that their blood pressure is now better (despite not having it checked), there is a clear opportunity for that allergy nurse to encourage that patient to seek further advice and have a positive impact on their health.

The specialist nurse cannot prescribe anti-hypertensives and solve the patient's hypertension but, approaching it from a public health point of view, they can encourage them to visit their doctor, and, if the patient seems receptive, explain the potentially devastating effects of uncontrolled hypertension and the need to take medication.

A basic veterinary-specific example would be if a cat attends a weight loss clinic with one of the nursing team, it would be remiss of that nurse not to mention something if they had noticed that the cat was very obviously suffering from dental disease.

A public health example in the context of One Health might be sought out for owners who admit to neglecting their own health. Consider the owner of a recently diagnosed diabetic cat who explains they are diabetic as well, but they do not bother with their medication. Surely this is an opportunity for a veterinary nurse who knows and understands diabetes to offer this owner some insight into the potential repercussions of neglecting their diabetes, as they support and educate them in the care of their cat.

Such interactions have the potential to support the care of the animal involved. Just as with the obese client continuing to share their takeaway with their overweight dog, the owner of a cat with diabetes who is careless with their own diabetic medication may be just as careless with their cat's health. It is entirely possible that a One Health approach may offer people a fresh approach, a new way of thinking about things and some inspiration to look after their own health a little better.

Not all veterinary nurses will feel confident in directly addressing issues associated with human health, even if the owner brings it up. However, basic signposting is easy and, critically, can be prepared in advance with a collection of robust, evidence-based resources on different topics. A leaflet, a website address, a clear signpost to contemporary evidence-based information – all have the potential to reach out and improve someone's health.

Perhaps an unexpected diagnosis of a health condition in an animal leads the owner to break down uncontrollably, and in between the tears they explain they feel overwhelmed by other areas of their life and this feels like the last straw. At this point, signposting may be helpful and a pre-researched resource invaluable to prevent a crisis emerging.

Making every contact count is simply about listening to people and considering whether there may be an opportunity to use transferable knowledge to support them to consider their own health and welfare.

It is important to note that making every contact count is not about adding something else to the 'to do' list on a busy day. It is an attitude. It is about the One Health approach; a broad concept of public health, considering the transferable information and skills and staying within the scope of practice but taking advantage of a potential opportunity. Finally, and most importantly, it is not about telling someone what to do or how to live their life.

6.3.4 Motivational Interviewing

A second technique equally applicable to veterinary nursing is the concept of motivational interviewing. Motivational interviewing (MI) suits a One Health public health approach for veterinary nurses. It has the clear benefit of allowing veterinary professionals to remain within their scope of practice while helping clients to help themselves with the aim of helping their pets. What is most relevant and critical about this technique is that it facilitates the use of the human–animal bond as an opportunity to support health decisions of the person.

MI uses a guiding conversational style, encouraging people to clarify their own motivations for healthcare-related actions which, within the context of veterinary, might be linked to their animal. There are patients whose animals might provide a stronger motivation to act than their medical team's instructions. A patient, anxious that she has been told she needs a coronary bypass operation, avoids the surgery, until her symptoms become so bad that it impacts on the distance she can walk her beloved dogs. Only then – when her animal's health is impacted – does she sign up for the surgery.

MI is a communication style with the aim of arranging conversations so that clients shift themselves towards change based on their own values and interests. Consider the obese owner of an equally obese dog who presents to the practice weight loss clinic. If exercise is mentioned in the context of exercise being good for all species, it allows the owner to consider the impact that taking the dog for more walks might have on themselves. Realizing that walking the dog more may help both their health and the dog's health may be a strong enough motivation to facilitate a change in their behaviour. Perhaps one of the most pertinent points about this is that such approaches are likely to be novel within human-centred healthcare.

Consider the topic of smoking cessation. An owner who smokes heavily will almost certainly have been told by medical healthcare professionals, probably on multiple occasions, that they need to stop smoking. However, it might only be when they are informed that their smoking is harming their animals that they realize they want to stop. Perhaps nobody has mentioned smoking in that context before?

The MI approach requires the use of open-ended questions, combined with attentive, reflective listening so that the professional in question can affirm and clarify what has been said. Once clarification has been sought, it is possible that self-motivational statements might transpire and those are important, as they demonstrate consideration of a reason to behave in a certain way – a motivation that critically has been realized independently as opposed to applied in a paternalistic way.

6.4 Skills for Public Health Nursing Projects

Nursing and public health share characteristics meaning that veterinary nurses may be ideally placed to instigate and develop public health projects within practice. It is important to realize that such projects will not always be easy. Public health often means tackling sensitive subjects and engagement with One Health can be apathetic at best and actively misunderstood at worst. To many it may be a new topic, as such demanding new ways of thinking, innovation, change – all concepts that can be deeply challenging, particularly in the context of a profession that is already busy and often stretched to the limit. Before embarking on such a project, consider the skills that are required for working in public health:

- Project management
- Research and knowledge
- Innovation
- Communication skills
- Assessment skills
- Technology

6.4.1 Project management

The science of managing projects has generated a vast amount of research and literature. Consequently, there is a wide range of frameworks and tools that can be used. It is important, particularly if the veterinary team involved are not familiar with public health, that a robust structure to educate and inform is used. It is preferable to use a framework that incorporates some evaluation and input from others. The 'Plan, Do, Study, Act' cycle is commonly used. Project sense-checking through the asking of pertinent questions is also useful. Examples include: what is the baseline? What parameters must be met for success? Where do we want to be at the end of this project? How will we get there? How will we know if we have got there?

6.4.2 Research and knowledge

As with all new projects, research to obtain high levels of background knowledge is critical for the credibility of the project and to establish if there are lessons to be learnt from other situations or experiences. The first place to start is usually with a literature review, then gathering local knowledge. Establishing local determinants of health, sometimes referred to on government websites as place-based assessments, provides a solid foundation on which to plan any interventions.

6.4.3   Innovation

By default, given that One Health is an emerging concept for many veterinary nurses, for those who wish to facilitate development of One Health, public health projects must be innovative. Equally important is situational awareness. It is important to take the time to check the context and to weigh up whether the time is right for discussions regarding new projects or ways of working. The first two weeks after a veterinary hospital has been taken over by a corporate is not the best time to ask people to work differently; a short-staffed team might also struggle, as might a team with a lot of inexperienced staff.

If it is judged that a team might be open to a public health project, the next task is to establish the scale of the project. Is it a small scale? An information board in reception linking through to public health messages about zoonosis or washing hands? Or is it the development of an advanced local project such as a veterinary outreach clinic targeting an area of the community known to struggle with significant social determinants of health, such as low income or poor housing?

One of the most innovative actions that VNs interested in public health can take is to reach out to local human-centred agencies, such as general practitioners (GPs) or charities, and ask, 'What can we do?' It might take some perseverance, but developing collaborative networks is the very essence of One Health and a direct example of public health in action.

6.4.4   Communication skills

Effective communication is at the heart of public health, regardless of the context. There is a need to be able to develop therapeutic relationships with owners, with other professionals and with colleagues. Templates and frameworks provide structure and guidance and there are many available to support concise and comprehensive communication.

6.4.5   Assessment skills

Advanced assessment skills combined with effective communication is essential to be able to evaluate an animal holistically and consider their health alongside and within the context of the health of their carer or owner. Again, as with the relevant communication skills, assessment frameworks are available to ensure that a holistic approach is taken and that critical assessment questions are not neglected.

6.4.6 Technology

The ability to use technology to support project working is essential. Data is held online regarding local social determinants of health. There is the potential for virtual meetings between agencies and stakeholders to facilitate effective time management and improve participation. Social media for networking, online collection of feedback, the use of apps to record health-related parameters – all offer opportunities to streamline working practice.

6.5   Guidelines for Public Health Projects in a Veterinary Nursing Context

There are five key points to consider when planning a public health or One Health project:

- Focus on the health of the population.
- Take the needs and priorities of the population into context.
- Ensure collaboration.
- Use a holistic approach.
- Always seek out evidence.

Firstly, the project should focus on the health of a population. The significant point here is that 'a population' is not necessarily 'the population'; it can be a local population, or a group of people with shared characteristics. The needs and priorities should be taken into context and used to guide the aims, objectives and content of the project. To ensure a positive One Health approach and offer support that allows individuals to remain within their scope of practice and still participate, there must be collaboration with other agencies, local GP surgeries, relevant charities or government groups. Work in this context should be holistic, incorporating a broad assessment and the knowledge and understanding that the health and wellbeing of an animal may well impact on the health and wellbeing of the owner. Finally, whatever its focus, the project should promote health, using evidence-based practices to ensure that professional codes of conduct are adhered to.

As an example, consider a veterinary nursing team wanting to offer support to the local homeless community, many members of which have pets who are also sleeping rough. Collaboration with local homelessness services allow a robust knowledge of the population – perhaps a joint exercise to offer support to the person as well as the animal. A holistic approach will ensure that the complexity of such a project is realized and anticipated. The community in question might be suspicious towards new initiatives, leading to a reluctance to engage with formal services, so novel ways of working might be suggested to suit the demographic of the population, such as visiting participants in the evening, offering informal 'meet and greet' sessions before the more formal health checks to begin to build therapeutic relationships. Finally, there is a need to ensure the services being offered are relevant and evidence based.

As well as formal specific project working, there are smaller individual approaches that can support public health within a veterinary nursing context and optimize encounters with owners from a health and wellbeing point of view.

6.5.1   One Health/public health project working

Signposting

Collaborate with local healthcare agencies to provide clients with information on subjects relevant to issues that are seen in practice, for example bereavement, domestic abuse, smoking cessation. There may also be the opportunity for interested members of staff to participate in specific specialist training to offer more advanced support for clients with specific health issues, for example clients of the practice with dementia.

Direct collaboration with public health campaigns

There is a huge amount of information that can be accessed to offer support and advice related to specific One Health, public health campaigns. Reception noticeboards or a social media monthly focus with associated links are potentially valuable tools to offer clients a different insight into familiar topics such as hand washing, vaccination or antibiotic resistance. In this case, a features list can be organized six months at a time, planning seasonally, selecting which agencies to link into. With some advanced planning, some social media posts can even be set up to send out automatically.

Offering CPD to forge public health links

Is there an issue that is particularly relevant to the health of the local community? Local social determinants of health might be a good starting point to plan a CPD/social or networking programme. The prevention of dog bites is a good example, where potentially, links with schools, playgroups and/or youth groups offers the chance for veterinary nurses to input positively into their local community.

Direct links with human-centred agencies

Consider a veterinary practice located in an area with high numbers of smokers. Perhaps the veterinary team are seeing these numbers reflected in the number of animals they see demonstrating signs consistent with being exposed to second-hand smoke. This is an excellent opportunity to reach out to the local GP; perhaps ask if there are any nurses in the practice who specialize in smoking cessation. They might be invited to share some of their experiences and offer some advice on how this potentially sensitive subject might be approached in a positive way.

6.5.2 Multidisciplinary team (MDT) working and collaborative practice

It is clear that considering the context of public health requires collaboration with others to optimize impact, knowledge and understanding. Effective public health in a One Health context relies on collaboration. Such collaboration may begin as sharing resources, and even the opportunity to 'see practice' with a member of the medical team and vice versa. Within the NHS, there are several nursing roles that might be of interest to veterinary nursing staff: intensive care, community nursing and tissue viability specialists are all ideally placed to offer valuable insights that might open up One Health opportunities.

Hints and tips for effective MDT working include the following.

- Preparation.
- Use project planning frameworks to structure collaborative working.
- Keep communication short and simple.
- Recognize and acknowledge the value of each team member's time and input.
- Keep all meetings running to time.
- Keep detailed records.
- Do not forget the clients.

Preparation

Before approaching colleagues, it is important to know exactly what the aims and objectives of the collaboration are. Once a dialogue is established, then those aims and objectives need to be discussed and agreed upon before a plan of action to achieve them can be put in place.

Using project planning frameworks to structure collaborative working

These tools ensure recognition of baseline, promote the use of evidence-based interventions and remind those involved to conduct a thorough evaluation in a timely manner. A popular example is the development of goals according to SMART goals (specific, measurable, achievable, relevant, timed).

Keeping communication short and simple

Consider using communication frameworks to streamline case presentations if being used to illustrate a point, or stimulate a discussion, for example SBAR (situation, background, assessment, recommendation).

Recognizing and acknowledging the value of each team member's time and input

Understand that One Health might not be top of everyone's agenda. Despite its importance, there are plenty of people not yet aware of its relevance; others may be keen to engage but are prevented by limited resource, so ensure that any time that is offered is appreciated.

Keeping all meetings running to time

If an agenda is set and agreed, it is important to stick to it. Late-running meetings can easily alienate people, especially if the tardiness is perceived to be due to a lack of organization.

Keeping detailed records

Ensure that minutes are taken, action points recorded and agreed upon before the meeting closes. Share any records to ensure that salient points have been recorded correctly.

Do not forget the clients

Consider including owners or clients as members of the multidisciplinary team. They have the potential to bring a novel point of view. In the UK's National Health Service, the 'expert patient' is a critical part of any service review, to ensure that feedback is gathered from the service users.

6.5.3   Benefits of collaboration

Collaboration is an essential part of any public health project within a One Health context: the very definition of One Health dictates a collaborative approach. As well as fulfilling the primary elements of One Health, there are several secondary benefits of collaboration.

- There is the potential for improved patient outcomes, using the human–animal bond. In particular for conditions such as obesity or diabetes that may affect both owner and animal, veterinary nurses have the power to educate owners about their animal's needs, and in turn, indirectly may be offering a novel way of discussing the owner's own health and wellbeing.
- Collaboration with clear communication can facilitate the development of shared goals and an agreed vision which is far more likely to succeed if all the stakeholders involved are engaged and in agreement.
- Understanding of each other's roles may be a huge advantage. Every role has its challenges and through sharing experiences, even attending different workplaces, those involved in the collaboration can learn and potentially empathize with others. No matter the species, healthcare work can be difficult and knowing that others can empathize can be comforting.

- Meetings, background research, clinical conversations and work-shadowing with multidisciplinary colleagues all have the potential to be valuable and free CPD which can be recorded and reflected on.
- When embarking on novel projects and concepts, it is important to consider them from all angles.

6.6 Potential Barriers to Public Health Working

While the benefits of working within a public health context have been discussed in this chapter there are also potential barriers to it being implemented. These include:

- Lack of knowledge
- Lack of resources
- Poor collaboration
- Difficulty in qualifying or quantifying results of a project
- Resistance to changing ways of working
- Belief that public health has no direct link to veterinary nursing

Lack of knowledge

Working in this context is relatively new to the veterinary profession. Background research is essential to ensure a high level of understanding to ensure that simple mistakes are not made and any dubious staff can be reassured and encouraged to participate.

Lack of resources

One Health might not be high on everyone's agenda. As such there will be some people who are keen to participate but struggling to release time to do so, or those whose organizations are constitutionally obliged to only work on projects that have been previously voted on by organizational stakeholders.

Poor collaboration

Ineffective or absent collaboration can lead to basic errors, which may undermine the entire project.

Difficulty quantifying results

A significant barrier to nurses working in a public health context, be it directly through human-centred nursing or veterinary nurses through the One Health context, is that it is difficult to quantify its impact. There may be some qualitative elements that can be collated, described and analysed, but it is critical to take the time at the start of each project to set recognizable goals with end points that allow evaluation and measure. Without such measures, members of any collaboration may quickly become disillusioned or overwhelmed by the magnitude of the topic.

Resistance to change

There may be resistance to changing ways of working. Change management is a well-studied discipline and there are numerous tools that may be enlisted.

Ignorance or misunderstanding

One of the biggest barriers to a public health project within the context of veterinary nursing is the belief that public health only concerns vets working in the food chain. The Veterinary Public Health Association (VPHA) is working hard to combat that attitude, listing the promotion of the role of the veterinary profession in public health at all levels as one of their key objectives.

6.7 On the Horizon – What Does the Future of Public Health in One Health Veterinary Nursing Look Like?

6.7.1 Veterinary social workers

The concept of a veterinary social worker marks a new paradigm of client and staff care. It represents a significant One Health collaboration with the potential to offer support and understanding to those who need it. While the model is almost exclusively found in the USA and Canada, it is certainly being talked about in the UK and there is an interest from some charity practices to begin to pilot such a role. There may be the potential to link in with social prescribing and support specific symptoms or conditions.

The role itself grew from acknowledging the strength of the human–animal bond and recognizing that there was a need to offer bereavement support to some people struggling with the loss of a much-loved pet. Other elements of the role may include supporting staff, helping those dealing with compassion fatigue or conflict in the workplace. The role is also responsible for signposting and organizing animal-assisted therapies and finally working with clients who might be affected by domestic violence, acknowledging that animals with non-accidental injuries are likely to have come from a household where others may have injuries from the perpetrator.

6.7.2 Inter-professional events and campaigns

While this chapter has emphasized how small-scale collaborations may benefit patients and the professionals involved, there is more scope for organizations to collaborate and begin to host partner events, potentially extending to campaigning. The dangers of passive smoking to animals were the topic of such collaboration between the Royal College of Nursing and the British Veterinary Nursing Association when they released a joint educational statement and press release on the subject. It was picked up by several television channels, radio stations and social media sites. Internationally it reached two continents with the opportunity for ongoing follow-up. Other partnerships that are planned include between human and veterinary critical care nurses and between nurses interested in wound management for all species. Both subjects have the potential for learning through sharing knowledge and experiences.

Collaboration may start between individuals but, just as with the potential for inter-professional events, if veterinary and human-centred healthcare agencies are more closely aligned there may be scope for cross-referrals. A veterinary practice with a strong working relationship with its local GP, for example, may feel happy referring a client there for some mental health support. Some mental health charities will accept referrals and offer a phone call to assess and support people. Such referrals do need permission from the animal's owner, but generally that can be done verbally, by asking them if they mind if someone gives them a call to see how they are getting on.

Finally, moving forward, it is important to aim high. Just as veterinary surgeons may sit on One Health boards and the government of One Health working groups, there is an argument that veterinary nurses should also be part of the conversation. VNs have the potential to bring a unique approach to public health in the One Health context, ensuring it remains practical, realistic and patient focused.

6.8 Questions for Further Discussion

1. How relevant is role modelling to public health? If a nurse is going to offer advice on obesity issues for an animal, does it matter if they themselves are grossly overweight?
2. Arguably it is easier for a VN to simply concentrate on the animal in a consultation rather than broaden the discussion to incorporate the opinions and values of the client on health and wellbeing. What advantages to the animal are there to having a broader discussion with the owner around their own health and wellbeing?
3. What is the most important skill required for working on a public health project in a One Health context? There may be several skills needed, but is there one in particular that, without it, the entire project would fall down?

6.9   Case Study: Lionel

Consider Lionel, a 55-year-old man with advanced prostate cancer, recovering from a recent pancreatectomy and receiving ongoing chemotherapy as a day patient. Before his cancer diagnosis he was a heavy smoker, daily drinker of alcohol and reliant on convenience food and take-away meals during the week while his wife was at work. He owns two dogs, who are by his own admission his 'pride and joy'. He has a good relationship with his wife, but she works long hours during the day; consequently he is alone for long periods of time. The dogs are up to date with their inoculations and do not have any chronic healthcare conditions. They are fed on a raw diet and both dogs are slightly overweight, although have both lost some weight recently.

Lionel's wife approaches you after you have removed a tick from one of their dogs in a nursing clinic consultation. She is extremely concerned about her husband interacting closely with the dogs, as she understands that the chemotherapy he is on suppresses his immune system and as such she is worried that the dogs will pass on a terrible disease.

What should you tell her?

Things to consider and discuss:

Dogs:

- Check vaccinations up to date.
- Give advice regarding safe handling of faeces.

Owners:

- Enquire whether her husband's recovery from his operation is far enough along to be able to explore his ability to walk the dogs and benefit from the exercise (advise seeking opinion of medical team before walking the dogs).
- Offer advice about use of live vaccines for the dogs according to data sheet of relevant medication.
- Give reassurance regarding risk being potentially offset by the level of company the dogs provide and the strength of the human–animal bond. Offer advice regarding allowing dogs to lick her husband, avoiding sleeping in same bed or sharing eating utensils, etc.
- Give reassurance that passing on of zoonotic disease is rare when sensible precautions are taken, e.g. handwashing.

Lionel's wife leaves the practice feeling reassured and happy that the dogs remain well placed to help her husband by providing stimulus for exercise and company while she is at work.

At the next oncology appointment Lionel's wife mentions her conversation with you to her specialist nurse. The specialist oncology nurse remarks that she often has questions from patients regarding pets and she has been meaning to write an information sheet on the topic. Lionel's wife puts her in touch with the practice team and together the human-centred nurse and veterinary nurse join forces to write a comprehensive guide to owning and enjoying pets while undergoing treatment for cancer. This is designed into a leaflet that is then kept available for people in the hospital and owners of animals at the vets.

Continued

> **Case Study** Continued.
>   The link created by working on this project remains in place and three months later a dialogue is opened as the specialist oncology nurse calls you to ask about provision for a pet when a patient has had to go into end-of-life care at a local hospice. You speak to a local animal charity and organize some emergency kennelling. When you report this back to the specialist nurse, she expresses her relief; the patient was refusing to leave until her dog was taken care of.
>
> **Consider:**
>
> - What are the key benefits of this collaboration?
> - Who benefits from this ongoing collaboration?
> - Are there any other elements of common conditions where further discussion between the two nurses might be of interest or even promote patient outcomes?
> - How can this chance encounter be used to increase the veterinary team's involvement in public health in their community?

References and Further Reading

Acheson, E.D. (1988) On the State of Public Health. *Public Health* 102(5), 431–437.

Evans, D., Coutsaftiki, D. and Fathers, C.P. (2017) *Health Promotion and Public Health for Nursing Students*, 3rd edn. Learning Matters (Sage Publications), London.

Linsley, P., Kane, R. and Owen, S. (2011) *Nursing for Public Health Promotion, Principles and Practice*. Oxford University Press, Oxford.

NICE (2022) *Making every contact count*. National Institute for Health and Care Excellence. Available at: https://stpsupport.nice.org.uk/mecc/index.html (accessed August 2022).

RCN (2019) *Working with dogs in healthcare settings*. Royal College of Nursing. Available at: https://www.rcn.org.uk/Professional-Development/publications/pub-007925 (accessed 1 May 2022).

RCVS (2014) *Code of Professional Conduct for Veterinary Nurses*. Royal College of Veterinary Nursing. Available at: http://www.rcvs.org.uk/advice-and-guidance/code-of-professional-conduct-for-veterinary-nurses/ (accessed 30 January 2022)

WHO (1999) *Definition of Veterinary Public Health*. World Health Organization, Geneva.

Environmental Sustainability in Veterinary Practice

7

Ellie West[1]*

[1]*Davies Veterinary Specialists, Hitchin; and Linnaeus*

7.1 Introduction to Environmentalism and Veterinary Healthcare

Humans are dependent upon our biosphere, but our activities have resulted in *'irreversible impacts as natural and human systems are pushed beyond their ability to adapt'* (IPCC, 2022). In 2021, medical and veterinary journals called for emergency action, saying that *'the science is unequivocal; a global increase of 1.5°C and the continued loss of biodiversity risks catastrophic harm to health that will be impossible to reverse'* (Atwoli *et al.*, 2021). Climate change alone is projected to cause 250,000 additional deaths globally per year between 2030 and 2050, with this healthcare crisis disproportionately affecting those people who have least contributed to its cause. In devastating irony, healthcare systems are also major contributors to ecological impacts. As described by Health Care Without Harm, *'if global healthcare were a country, it would be the 5th largest greenhouse gas emitter on the planet'* (HCWH, 2019).

We have been *'mortgaging the health of future generations to realise economic and development gains in the present'* (Whitmee *et al.*, 2015). Tackling these ecosystem crises may be our greatest global health opportunity, by moving towards a vision of healthcare which manages any harms we cause and adapts to the challenges that we face (Watts *et al.*, 2015). In this chapter, we explore three areas: (i) the links between veterinary healthcare and ecosystems; (ii) how registered veterinary nurses (RVNs) can practise more sustainably; and (iii) how we can influence and lead in our wider communities.

7.2 Linking Ecosystems and Veterinary Healthcare

Nature provides us with goods and services (Table 7.1) that are essential for our wellbeing but are not often included in calculations of national wealth.

*Email: ellie.west@vetspecialists.co.uk

© CAB International 2023. *One Health for Veterinary Nurses and Technicians*
(eds R. Jones and A. Jeffery)
DOI: 10.1079/9781789249477.0007

Table 7.1. Ecosystems services. (Adapted from WRI, 2005; IPBES, 2019.)

Ecosystems services	Examples of services
Provisioning	Food, fresh water, fuels, genetic resources and pharmaceuticals
Regulating	Air, soil and water quality, pollination, climate stability, disease control, and natural hazards mitigation such as flood control
Cultural	Recreation, education, mental and physical health, social, spiritual, inspiration and scientific activities
Indirect supporting	Soil formation and nutrient cycling

Nature is particularly vulnerable to overuse where resources are shared, silent, invisible, or mobile (Dasgupta, 2021).

Since 1970, a global decline has occurred in 14 of 18 Nature's services (IPBES, 2019). The Planetary Boundaries model outlines key biophysical processes which define a safe operating space for humanity on Earth, and by 2022 we had crossed five of the nine boundaries: climate change, biodiversity loss, nitrogen and phosphate cycles and novel entities (plastics and chemicals) (Fig. 7.1) (Persson *et al.*, (2022). These boundaries are interlinked; for example, reducing functional biodiversity leaves ecosystems more vulnerable to climate change. Measures to protect one boundary may also have unintended consequences for another.

The Millennium Sustainable Development Goals (SDGs) are a United Nations (UN) framework for a One Health approach. These are a set of 17 targets to mutually benefit and grow economies, society and Nature (UN, 2021). The SDGs demonstrate the depth of interconnection between the health of human and natural ecosystems; indeed, we are all dependent on One Health. There is a growing body of evidence on the environmental impacts of veterinary healthcare, but also on how ecosystem changes will impact our ability to provide healthcare. In this section, we focus on the triple threat of climate change, resource use and biodiversity loss.

7.2.1   The science of climate change for veterinary practices

The Earth's atmospheric carbon dioxide (CO_2) concentration was stable for 10,000 years, acting alongside other greenhouse gases (GHGs) as insulation against extreme temperatures. Since the industrial era in the 19th century, fossil fuel combustion has exponentially increased atmospheric CO_2 concentrations to 415 ppm, raising the average global surface temperature by 1.1°C. Temperature rises are projected to exceed 1.5°C during the 21st century, with the severity of harm to humans, animals and ecosystems increasing with temperatures. We may also see non-linear tipping events such as loss of a year-round northern ice sheet (which reflects heat and insulates the oceans) or

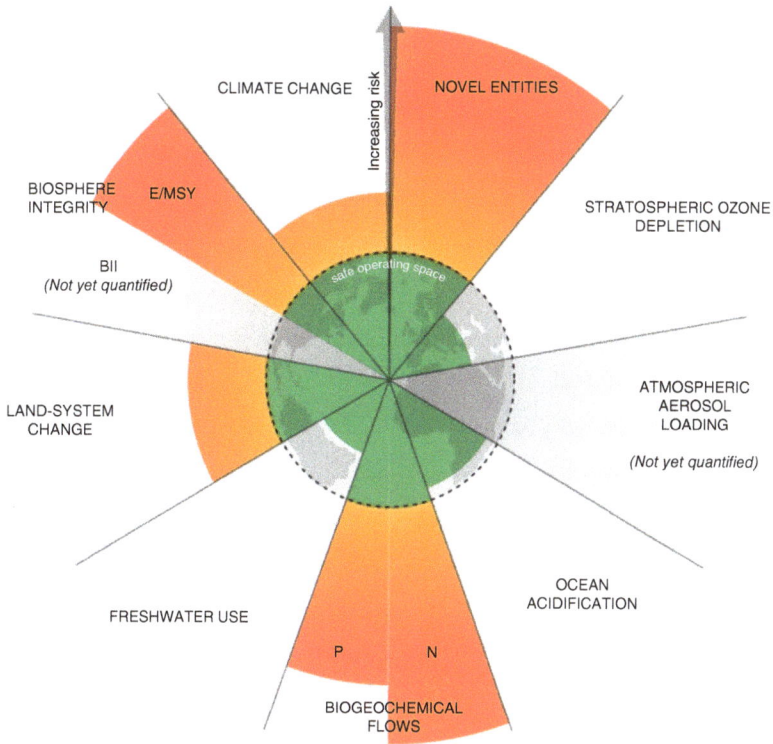

Fig. 7.1. The Planetary Boundaries model. Inner green indicates safe operating spaces; orange represents high risk zones for humanity to operate within. BII, biodiversity intactness index, or functional diversity; E/MSY, genetic diversity; N, nitrogen; P, phosphorus. (Credit: J. Likrantz/Azote, based on Steffen *et al.*, 2015; available for use under license CC BY 4.0)

melting of permafrost (currently storing the GHG methane) (IPCC, 2022). In the UK, high-risk events for humans and animals include heat stress, flooding, water shortages, reduced food production and emerging diseases (Defra, 2017; Lacetera, 2018). Globally, health morbidities and mortalities include dehydration, infections, mental health outcomes, allergies, cardiovascular and pulmonary diseases (Atwoli *et al.*, 2021).

The ability of individual GHGs to cause global heating depends on four factors: (i) their atmospheric lifetime; (ii) how well they absorb heat (radiative forcing); (iii) their range of action (absorption wavelength); and (iv) the total amount released (for example, if a particular clinical effect requires a higher dose of a less potent drug). Individual molecules are compared by their Global Warming Potential (GWP_{100}), but different amounts of different molecules can be compared (with CO_2 as a GHG) using CO_2 equivalency (mass $\times$ GWP_{100} = $kgCO_2e$); so nitrous oxide has high carbon equivalency for clinical use given its high GWP_{100} and low potency. Table 7.2 illustrates a comparison of anaesthetic agents regularly used in the veterinary clinic.

Carbon equivalents from an individual product or process are calculated using life cycle analysis (LCA), which calculates all emissions from material extraction to disposal (cradle-to-grave). For instance, this can inform us that a medical cataract operation performed in one country or another produces 6 or 130 $kgCO_2e$, despite similar clinical outcomes (Sherman *et al.*, 2020). An LCA of the alpha-2 agonist drugs xylazine and dexmedetomidine found that either 20 or 3000 $kgCO_2e$ per kilogram of active pharmaceutical ingredient, respectively, were produced (Parvatker *et al.*, 2019). LCA also identifies carbon hotspots. Most emissions for pharmaceuticals result from solvent and energy usage during production, drug packaging and sterilization (Jeswani and Azapagic, 2020). In the future, carbon information may be available to veterinary professionals to guide our choices by environmental impact alongside clinical outcomes.

7.2.2 How veterinary clinics use resources

Earth Overshoot Day marks the annual date when humanity's 'ecological footprint', or raw material use, exceeds the 'biocapacity' for production; in 2021 it was 29 July. Increasing consumption is driven by global trends such as urbanization, but our consumption intensity is also increasing. Whilst the population doubled over the past 50 years, the global economy quadrupled. Supplies of critical resources are at risk: 23% of land has reduced productivity due to environmental degradation (IPBES, 2019). Over time, depleting natural capital increases vulnerability to climate events, which negatively impacts health and wellbeing and exacerbates conflict.

Veterinary clinics use diverse raw materials, including plastics and rare-earth elements. Operating theatres are particularly resource-intensive, with single-use devices common due to concerns around infectious and hazardous

Table 7.2. Atmospheric characteristics of volatile anaesthetic agents (Campbell and Pierce, 2015; McGain *et al.*, 2020). See also section 7.3.1.

	Carbon dioxide	Sevoflurane	Isoflurane	Nitrous oxide
Atmospheric lifetime (years)	74	1.1	3.2	110
Global warming potential over 100 years (GWP_{100})	1	130	510	265
Carbon equivalents ($kgCO_2e$)[a]		49 $kgCO_2e$/ 250 ml	190 $kgCO_2e$/ 250 ml	0.56 $kgCO_2e$/litre
Minimum alveolar concentration in dogs (%)		2.3	1.3	188–222

[a]$kgCO_2e$ = unit of carbon footprints measured in kilograms of carbon dioxide equivalent

materials. LCAs for medical textiles and equipment also report impacts such as water, land and resource use, toxicity, eutrophication, chemical oxygen demand, ozone depletion and air pollution, including particulate matter and volatile emissions.

For the RVN, the mission should be to provide quality healthcare with reduced use of resources, creating functional circular economies to eliminate waste, circulate materials, and regenerate Nature. Experiences of reusable systems such as oxygen generators and washable surgical textiles highlight the benefits of supply-chain resilience and financial savings to maintaining quality healthcare.

7.2.3   Biodiversity and veterinary healthcare

Current extinction rates are hundreds to thousands of times higher than background rates (Dasgupta, 2021). International reports find that one million plant, animal and insect species are threatened with extinction and populations of vertebrate species declined by 58% over 40 years (IPBES, 2019; WWF, 2020). The main drivers of biodiversity loss are land- and sea-use change, over-exploitation of species, climate change, pollution, invasive species and disease.

We need biodiversity for healthcare; around 75% of global food crops rely on animal pollination, and a similar proportion of anti-cancer drugs originate from Nature (IPBES, 2019). Intact ecosystems provide resilience from environmental shocks; for example, coastal flooding from storms is reduced by mangrove swamps. Preventing habitat fragmentation may also reduce zoonotic spillover and emergence of infectious diseases (Glidden *et al.*, 2021).

Pollution is an emerging cause of human health problems, with air pollution causing 16% of all deaths globally (Landrigan *et al.*, 2018). Pharmaceutical and chemical pollution is a rising problem; for instance, manufacture of medical textiles contributes to microplastics and chemical pollution and over 25% of global rivers contain medical pharmaceutical residues (PRs) at concentrations unsafe for aquatic organisms, or of concern for antimicrobial resistance (HCWH, 2022a,b; Wilkinson *et al.*, 2022). The main pathways for PRs to reach the environment are as active metabolites (30–90% of oral pharmaceuticals are excreted as active substances in urine and faeces), improper disposal by consumers, and wastewater from manufacture sites (EC, 2018). The impact of PRs depends on a variety of factors, including environmental concentration, frequency of exposures, drug interactions, bioavailability and species (EC, 2018; Bennett and Weeks, 2021). Cumulative ecologic and public health impacts of mixed pollutants are poorly understood.

Authorizations for veterinary pharmaceuticals include environmental risk assessments, although these are focused on food-producing species and are limited for companion animal medications. There is ongoing research into the bioavailability, sources and impacts of veterinary PRs. Environmental risks in

---

Box 7.1. An RVN's role in pharmaceutical stewardship.

Most RVNs will be aware of the need for drug stewardship programmes due to the global One Health threat posed by antimicrobial resistance (see Chapter 2, The Human–Animal–Environment Interface; and Chapter 5, Communicable Diseases). However, pharmaceuticals can also cause ecological harm due to carbon emissions, resource extraction and pollution.

Medicines and chemicals make up 20% of healthcare's carbon footprint. To make 1 kg of the antibiotic vancomycin, 57 kgCO$_2$e are emitted, mostly from energy use, and 585 kg of materials is used, predominantly water (Ponder and Overcash, 2010). Ecosystems are also affected by pharmaceutical residues, which acutely and chronically impair the growth, reproduction and immune function of non-target organisms (EC, 2018). Additional pressures result from climate change (causing ocean acidification and extreme weather events) and other pollutants.

Veterinary products make up 3% of EU pharmaceutical sales, with antimicrobials, vaccines and parasiticides being the highest (EC, 2018). Whilst the majority of veterinary pharmaceuticals are used in the food-producing sector, there is a clear ecological case for promoting responsible pharmaceutical stewardship in clinics, which RVNs can support in a number of ways. These include raising awareness of the need for pharmaceutical stewardship amongst owners (including farm clients), veterinary surgeons and other professionals, by promoting infection control measures (see section 7.3.4), by focusing on pharmaceutical waste segregation and management (see section 7.3.3) and by empowering owners to provide preventive care for pets (see section 7.4.2).

---

specific exposure scenarios are highlighted for anti-parasiticides, antibiotics and some endocrine-disrupters (Bártíková *et al.*, 2016; EC, 2018; Mahefarisoa *et al.*, 2021; Perkins *et al.*, 2021). Guidance from the European Medicines Agency is under review, including labelling of the environmental risk of medicinal products and indexing based on persistence, bioaccumulation and toxicity of drugs.

7.3 Environmental Sustainability in the Clinic

The 2019 COVID pandemic generated rapid transformative change and may have improved attitudes towards conserving Nature and resources, reuse innovations, reduced travel, remote access to care and a focus on preventive medicine (McGain *et al.*, 2021). Around half of pet owners said they would pay more for veterinary treatment with reduced environmental impact (Deluty *et al.*, 2021).

By 2022, a sector-endorsed Greener Veterinary Practice Checklist was launched by VetSustain, with a vet carbon calculator which can be used alongside medical resources such as the Greener Practice Network and GP carbon calculator (RCGP, 2022). The Royal College of Veterinary Surgeons (RCVS) has an Environment and Sustainability Working Party which integrated sustainability into the Practice Standards Scheme framework in 2022. Consensus statements and resources from NHS England and the Association of Anaesthetists lay out responsibilities and pathways to net zero carbon emissions. Open-access journals such as the *Lancet Planetary Health* are driving literacy, whilst peer-support and online practical guidance is available from groups such as the Royal College of Medicine's Climate Change series, the Royal College of General Practioners' Green Impact for Health Toolkit, UK Healthcare Alliance on Climate Change, the Centre for Sustainable Healthcare and Health Care Without Harm. The Royal College of Nurses recently published its guide to Sustainable Nursing Practice, and the international NurSuS project provides free training in sustainability literacy and competency.

Of the various healthcare sectors, hospital care causes 40% of the carbon footprint (NHS, 2021a). A veterinary clinic generates carbon emissions as part of its direct operational (Scope 1 and 2) and indirect (Scope 3) activities. For NHS England, Scope 1 and 2 account for 24% of emissions, with the remainder due to Scope 3 emissions, which include the supply chain for pharmaceuticals, medical equipment and commissioned services. Table 7.3 provides conversion factors to calculate a veterinary clinic's carbon emissions.

Thiel *et al.* (2018) suggested that carbon emissions from one surgery (a laparoscopic hysterectomy) can be reduced by 80%, with 50% of these savings resulting from minimizing and reusing surgical equipment, and 25% from replacing desflurane and N_2O as anaesthetic agents. Only 5% of emissions were saved by minimizing waste (by recycling and reusable textiles), although these actions will reduce procurement emissions and disposal impacts. Next, we discuss key opportunities for RVNs to reduce the environmental impacts in their practice.

7.3.1 Anaesthetic agents

Anaesthesia is an energy, resource and carbon-intense event (Jones and West, 2019). Medical anaesthetists agree that whilst patient safety should not be

Table 7.3. Carbon conversion factors for common sources of emissions (Rizan *et al.*, 2021; UK Government, 2022).

Scope	Category	Emissions source	Conversion factor (units)
1	Energy	Mains gas in 2022	0.18219 kgCO$_2$e/kWh
1	Transport	Average UK passenger car – unknown fuel – 2022	0.27465 kgCO$_2$e/mile
1	Anaesthetic gases	See Table 7.2	
2	Electricity	National grid in 2022	0.19338 kgCO$_2$e/kWh
3	Waste	High temperature incineration	1074 kgCO$_2$e/tonne
		Recovery (energy-from-waste)	172 kgCO$_2$e/tonne
		Food: anaerobic digestion	9 kg CO$_2$e/tonne
3	Water		0.149 kgCO$_2$e/m^3

compromised by sustainable anaesthetic practices, healthcare systems and an-aesthesia providers should reduce their contribution to global warming (White *et al.*, 2022).

Anaesthetic agents (AAs) are potent GHGs. Active scavenging systems (and passive systems without incineration) release AAs unchanged into the atmosphere, where they may contribute to two-thirds of a medical surgery's $562\ kgCO_2e$ footprint (Thiel *et al.*, 2018). Recapture systems which could enter anaesthetic agents into a circular economy are not yet commercially available. Whilst only 2% of NHS England's carbon emissions result from AAs, they are disproportionately impactful, due to absorption of heat within an 'atmospheric window' where few naturally occurring GHGs act. Medical guidance has recently been published for addressing pollution from inhalational anaesthetics (Devlin-Hegedus *et al.*, 2022).

The RCVS defines the RVN as '*the most suitable person to assist a veterinary surgeon to monitor and maintain anaesthesia*'. RVNs are often responsible for choosing anaesthetic consumables and equipment, whereas the responsibility for drug choice, delivery technique and dose rests with the veterinary surgeon.

Perioperative choices

Shorter durations of anaesthesia, efficient workflows and (where appropriate) using sedative/injectable agents or regional anaesthetic techniques will reduce AA consumption. Improved analgesia also stabilizes the plane of anaesthesia, reducing the need for higher fresh gas flows (FGF) to achieve rapid increases in anaesthetic depth.

Lower-flow anaesthesia

The amount of AA used is directly proportional to the FGF and vaporizer setting. Low-flow anaesthesia (reducing FGF closer to metabolic oxygen re-quirements of around 10 ml/kg/min) will reduce GHG impacts, although it can result in hypoxic gas delivery and accidental patient awareness. Independent of the breathing system, reducing FGFs below 1 l/min is not recommended without suitable experience, monitoring (capnography, end-tidal agent and inspired oxygen concentrations) and rotameters and vaporizers capable of precision delivery. Higher FGFs may be needed for equipment-related inefficiencies, including gas sampling and leaks; regular leak testing and machine/pipe/manifold maintenance should be performed. Capnography reduces equipment errors such as leaks, exhausted CO_2 absorbent or disconnections.

FGFs above the metabolic oxygen requirement are often used. For circle rebreathing systems (with CO_2 absorbent), excess FGF denitrogenates the body at the start of anaesthesia and speeds changes in anaesthetic depth; FGF may therefore be reduced once anaesthetic depth is stable. However, for non-re-breathing systems, the excess FGF primarily prevents rebreathing of CO_2 during inspiration. This means a capnograph can be used to optimize FGFs to

Box 7.2. Lower-flow anaesthesia

Modelling of lower-flow anaesthesia in a veterinary clinic shows the potential for a 63% reduction in GHG emissions by limiting FGF to 1 l/min using appropriate breathing systems (McMillan, 2021). When using isoflurane 2%, a reduction in FGF from 2 to 1 l/min halves the carbon emissions from 9.5 to 4.7 kgCO$_2$e/hour (Pierce, 2015). The annual UK carbon footprint is around 7 tCO$_2$e/person. Carbon choices include recycling all domestic waste or eating a plant-based diet, saving 0.2–0.8 tCO$_2$e/year, or for the veterinary nurse reducing FGF by 25% saves 3.5 tCO$_2$e/year (from 3 l/min, assuming 2% isoflurane and 4 hours of anaesthesia per working day) (Wynes and Nicholas, 2017).

In 2021 the Linnaeus Veterinary Group created the We Go for Lower Flow campaign, which comprised a Quality Improvement initiative to deliver anaesthetic monitors capable of capnography, with specialist-led support for lower-flow anaesthesia, including posters, educational webinars, live teaching forums and a quiz (West, 2021; Linnaeus, 2022). Co-benefits of using capnography included reduced occupational exposure through identification of equipment leaks, financial savings, and improved quality of care, including for management of cardiopulmonary arrest.

The main barriers to reducing FGFs were a lack of equipment capable of precision delivery and confidence in using capnography. The risks of lower-flow anaesthesia included unstable depths of anaesthesia, if the FGF was reduced too early after anaesthetic induction.

The principles of We Go for Lower Flow are as follows.

General cautions

- Any changes in anaesthetic protocol should be within the veterinary professional's ability and the equipment available. Specialist advice should be sought if needed.
- Vaporizers and rotameters should be capable of accurately delivering gases at 1 l/min.
- Excessive dead space may also cause rebreathing of CO$_2$ with any system.

Circle rebreathing systems (with CO$_2$ absorbent):

- Patient weight over 5–10 kg (check with manufacturer) and up to 100kg
- *Fresh gas flow:*
  - Use oxygen at 2 l/min for 5–10 min at the start and end of anaesthesia, when moving between systems and when changing anaesthetic depth
  - Reduce FGF to 1 l/min once anaesthetic depth is stable
- *Cautions:*
  - Monitor anaesthetic depth closely due to the 'dilution effect' and be prepared to use injectable anaesthesia for rapid changes in anaesthetic depth. Emptying the rebreathing bag can reduce 'dilutional' effects and avoid increases in FGF.
  - Exhausted CO$_2$ absorbent or faulty valves may also cause rebreathing of CO$_2$.

Non-rebreathing systems:

- Patient weight under 5–10 kg (check with manufacturer)
- *Fresh gas flow calculation:*

Continued

Box 7.2. Continued.

- Use a capnograph to adjust the FGF to just prevent rebreathing of CO_2
- Or use Mapleson A systems (e.g. mini-lack) with 200 ml/kg/min and Mapleson D, E and F systems (e.g. T-piece variants) at 500 ml/kg/min

Between 2020 and 2021, Linnaeus saw a reduction in normalised anaesthetic gas purchases by around 25%. This work suggests that by building awareness and providing appropriate support and equipment, veterinary teams can effectively reduce anaesthetic gas consumption. The resources are now available online (Linnaeus, 2022)

---

just prevent CO_2 rebreathing with non-rebreathing systems only, as described in Box 7.2.

Choice of drug

AAs have varying environmental impacts (see Table 7.2) with the most harmful having high GWP_{100}, longer atmospheric persistence and/or lower potency (requiring more drug for clinical effect). Of the most harmful agents, N_2O can be avoided with well-planned analgesic protocols, and desflurane is not commonly used.

Despite its lower potency, sevoflurane is around 50% less carbon-intensive than isoflurane (assuming lower carbon manufacture pathways) due to its lower GWP_{100} (Hu *et al.*, 2021). Sevoflurane products currently carry a licensing warning to avoid long-duration, low-flow anaesthesia, due to a nephrotoxic molecule called compound A forming from an interaction with CO_2 absorbents. No reports of harm exist in clinical veterinary anaesthesia and there is debate as to the medical significance, but there is no published consensus as yet on the safety of sevoflurane for prolonged low-flow anaesthesia in animals (Kennedy *et al.*, 2019).

Total intravenous anaesthesia (TIVA)

Propofol and alfaxalone carry UK licences for maintaining anaesthesia in dogs and cats, although the dose and duration of anaesthesia are limited depending on the manufacturer and product. Early studies suggested that TIVA could reduce carbon emissions to 1% of inhalational anaesthetic emissions, although recapture technology (once available) could produce equivalent emissions from propofol or recaptured sevoflurane anaesthesia (McGain *et al.*, 2020; Hu *et al.*, 2021). Propofol is considered as low environmental risk, due to limited use, despite its persistence and aquatoxicity. TIVA also uses plastics and energy for delivery, although bioplastics and renewable electricity may be available. Finally, TIVA has technical and clinical challenges that limit its practical use.

7.3.2 Sustainable procurement

Sustainable procurement defines how we meet business supply needs whilst driving positive impacts on a life cycle basis for ecosystems, pets, owners and communities. Goal 12 of the UN's Sustainable Development Goals is 'Responsible Consumption and Production', and targets include reducing material footprints, increasing reuse and recycling, and sustainable procurement policies.

With 60% of NHS England's carbon footprint originating in its supply chain, many organizations are engaging with their suppliers as part of their net zero carbon targets. Key sustainability criteria for suppliers can be defined in a Code of Conduct. Depending on the organization's environmental priorities, this may include accreditations, net zero targets, renewable electricity, lower carbon transport, waste and water reduction, and/or biodiversity projects. For example, consolidating deliveries, reusing tote boxes, taking back packaging and local sourcing can support a practice's sustainability targets. Engaging with suppliers has the wider benefit of improving standards across the sector.

For veterinary staff, the first step is to **buy less**. Focus areas should include the following.

- Purchasing for **longevity and reuse**. Setting up staff swap-shops for domestic items encourages a reuse culture.
- **Streamlining processes** by reviewing redundancy in disposable kits. Thiel *et al.* (2018) found that minimizing material use and selecting reusable surgical instruments created 50% carbon savings for each procedure.
- Using **non-pharmaceutical adjunctive treatments** where appropriate. For certain conditions, such as diabetes and osteoarthritis, patient outcomes may improve with nutritional or physical therapies (see section 7.4.2).

Secondly, **reducing pharmaceutical waste** can be supported by:

- **Robust stock control**, which prevents wastage from over-ordering, slow-moving or out-of-date stock.
- **Careful prescribing** with exact amounts, shorter starter packs where appropriate, and with clearly labelled disposal methods.
- Promoting **responsible pharmaceutical stewardship** (see Chapter 5, Communicable Diseases; see also section 7.2.3).
- **Oral prescription** over non-enteral routes where appropriate: a 1 g intravenous paracetamol dose produces 100 times more carbon emissions than the same oral dose (Hayes and Froom, 2022).
- **Auditing waste** to identify opportunities for streamlining; around 50% of prepared propofol goes unused (McGain *et al.*, 2020).

Thirdly, where disposable resources are necessary to maintain quality of care, seek available **eco-friendly options**:

- **Streamlined material content** – lower plastic syringes, recycled content (e.g. Elizabethan collars, bin bags, paper products).
- **Plant-based solutions** – dispensing in paper bags, plant-based disposable aprons, UN-approved cardboard pharmaceutical bins, wood-based cat litter.

- **Avoid harmful materials and chemicals** – find alternatives to PVC and polystyrene. Be aware of harmful chemicals (HCWH, 2018).
- **Take-back of unused medications** – drug amnesties encourage clients to return unused or out-of-date medications.
- **Eco-labels** – environmental product declarations support green claims. The website www.ecolabelindex.com provides guidance.

All UK public health systems must use their buying power to generate social and environmental benefits. Tools include a Flexible Framework for Sustainable Procurement which focuses on leadership, communication, processes, engaging suppliers and measuring outcomes. Healthcare Without Harm (HCWH 2022a,b) has created examples of procurement criteria for medical products. The British Medical Association's Ethical Procurement for Health workbook also addresses human rights issues, which are more prevalent for low-cost, high-volume items such as medical gloves.

7.3.3   Waste management and disposal

Waste volumes from veterinary clinics could increase with global pet populations. UK medical hospitals produce 3.3 kg waste daily per patient, with correlations between higher quality systems and increased waste. Due to its hazardous nature and depending on available disposal options, medical waste has environmental impacts ranging from GHG emissions (incineration and landfill) to microplastics, chemical leachate from landfills, air pollutants from incineration, and aquatoxicity from drugs and chemical release (Kenny and Priyadarshini, 2021).

Legal controls

UK waste regulations are designed to protect public health and the environment. The Environmental Protection Act 1990 mandates a duty of care for everyone in the waste management chain. All healthcare waste must be documented, segregated (not mixed), stored, transported and disposed of in accordance with the European Waste Catalogue (EWC) coding system. It is the waste producer's responsibility to ensure that waste contractors are appropriately permitted. All veterinary professionals should receive waste management training.

Veterinary clinic waste falls into two broad categories: domestic waste (not contaminated), and healthcare waste (contaminated with clinical materials). Some types of waste are sub-classified as hazardous (e.g. infectious material, sharps, cytotoxic/cytostatics), meaning tighter controls and higher costs. In general, domestic waste may be landfilled, segregated for recycling, or incinerated with energy capture, whilst healthcare waste is sent for heat sterilization or high-temperature incineration depending on the level of risk. Offensive waste may also be landfilled or (for limited sub-types with appropriate permitting) recycled. Differences exist between the devolved UK nations (BVA, 2011; Department of Health, 2013; West *et al.*, 2020).

Reducing waste impacts in veterinary practice

The cornerstones of the waste hierarchy are to reduce, reuse and recycle, with rethinking and researching as newer additions. A waste audit will identify what is wasted and what could be better segregated in your clinic.

1. REDUCE   Operating rooms produce 25% of hospital waste, with most generated before the patient arrives, including sterile packets, rigid containers, and drape wraps. Opportunities include:

- Pre-packed kits
- Single sterile bagging for low cost, soft consumables
- Smaller volumes of prepared drugs or pre-filled (longer-lasting) syringes
- Water distillers to replace bottled sterile water for autoclaves
- Remanufactured or refillable print cartridges with plant-based inks; refillable pens
- Regular maintenance to prolong equipment lifespan; redistribution and donation of functional (and serviceable) equipment
- Electronic billing and administration systems (see section 7.3.8)

2. REUSE   Reusable medical equipment and textiles have less environmental impacts than single-use options. Reusables reduce carbon emissions by 66% for textiles and 84% for anaesthetic equipment, whilst compared with disposables, reusable gowns reduce waste by 84% (Overcash, 2012; Vozzola *et al.*, 2020).

Barriers to reuse include reprocessing facilities and logistics (including tracking, packaging and laundry), liabilities resulting from malfunction of single use items, and infection control (see section 7.3.4). Reuse must not increase infection risks (which carry a carbon cost) or harm. For instance, rinsing pharmaceutical containers could cause waterway pollution; however, disposing of pharmaceutical waste in regulated reusable containers reduces carbon emissions by 84% alongside lower plastic production and incineration (Grimmond *et al.*, 2021). Clinical reuse opportunities include:

- Metal surgical instrument cases to replace blue polypropylene wrap
- Textiles, including warming blankets, scrub hats, drapes, gowns and Type 2r masks – seek natural fibres, lower-impact chemicals, low-impact laundry and recyclability (HCWH, 2022b)
- Rechargeable batteries
- Rubber matting (in kennels)
- Washable incontinence pads
- Wipe-clean grooming aprons
- Reusable diathermy mats

3. RECYCLING   Up to 60% of anaesthetic waste can be recycled (Jones and West, 2019) but segregation compliance relies on having the right containers in the right places. Being prepared at the beginning of procedures allows recyclables to be separated before contamination. Recycling opportunities include:

- Printer cartridges and batteries
- Unrepairable metal instruments and fabrics
- Recyclable plastics
- Crystalloid containers can be recycled only if they are not contaminated with infectious materials, cytotoxic/cytostatic or pharmaceutical agents, and any sharps are removed. Practices should check with waste contractors for appropriate licences before recycling offensive waste

4. RETHINK   As waste producers, practices must segregate according to the Waste Hierarchy, which prioritizes more environmentally friendly options. Opportunities for alternative choices include:

- **Waste training** – to promote correct segregation
- **Alternative disposal** – sending food waste to anaerobic digestion rather than landfill reduces carbon emissions from 627 to 9 $kgCO_2e/t$ and creates biogas and fertilizer (UK Government, 2021)
- **Biodegradable plastics** – only beneficial if waste streams are landfilled, although may produce less toxic incineration products. Labelling should differentiate biodegradable from compostable or industrially compostable
- **Circular economy thinking** – seeking options to treat waste as a raw resource for creation of new materials

5. RESEARCH   Further research may establish the best available technique to mitigate environmental harms over the lifecycle of a product or drug. For instance, surgical treatment of reflux in humans carries a higher initial carbon cost than medical management, but produces lower carbon emissions after the 9th year (Gatenby, 2011). The National Institute for Health Research's carbon reduction guidelines assess '*the environmental impact of proposed interventions ... alongside clinical and cost effectiveness*'.

7.3.4   Infection control

Infection control is predominantly an RVN-led activity to reduce the risk of pathogen transmission, thereby reducing pet and staff infections, but it will also reduce resource and chemical use from treatment of infections. Infection control guidelines for veterinary practice are available (Stull *et al.*, 2018), alongside standards within the RCVS Practice Standards Scheme.

Hand hygiene is a frequently overlooked but key part of infection control. One study found that '*disposable medical devices and attire in the operating theatre do not mitigate the infectious risk to the patients but ... it appears that pathogen transmission ... is mainly due to the lack of hand hygiene'* (Reynier *et al.*, 2021). The Royal College of Nurses runs a Glove Awareness campaign to streamline non-sterile glove use, since these can potentially raise infection transmission by preventing hand hygiene and contributing to user dermatitis.

Veterinary clinics use a range of chemicals for surface infection control, depending on the intended use of the area or item. Cleaning is the removal of foreign material from objects and is normally accomplished using water with detergents or enzymatic products. Disinfection kills or inactivates pathogenic microorganisms (with sterilization additionally destroying spores) but requires concurrent cleaning to be effective. Properties of an ideal disinfectant include broad-spectrum activity (against bacteria, viruses, yeasts and fungi), rapid action, non-toxic, easy to apply without protective equipment, non-corrosive, stable and effective as one-stage cleaner-disinfectants. Overuse may result in disinfectant-resistant pathogens. Some cleaning chemicals are linked to human health issues, including ethylene oxide, glutaraldehydes and quaternary ammoniums (Rutala and Weber, 2021). Risks are outlined in product Safety Data Sheets, alongside manufacturers' recommendations for any personal protective equipment (usually single-use plastics). The European WIDES database and US Safer Choice program categorize chemicals by health and environmental safety using Globally Harmonized System hazard codes.

In the UK, veterinary disinfectants are governed by the Biocidal Products Regulations, with testing chemicals against veterinary pathogens currently allowing classification as Product Type 3. A Defra-approved disinfectant must be used in the case of notifiable disease outbreaks.

Approaches to reducing the environmental impact of infection control include:

- **Streamlining use of higher-impact chemicals by zoning** – for instance, an operating theatre requires more intense cleaning than a staff room.
- **Switching to lower-impact chemicals** where possible within current regulatory and quality requirements. Guidance on choosing safer healthcare disinfectants is available (HCWH, 2020).
- **Careful disposal of chemicals and packaging** following manufacturers' instructions.
- **Use of non-chemical cleaning methods where appropriate** – microfibre cloths can be used with water for cleaning; ideally those with certified cleaning ability, low microfibre shedding and recycled plastic content. Filters for washing machines can reduce microplastic contamination. Steam cleaners are used in the NHS, but require plastic consumables and electricity. Ultraviolet-light sterilizing systems are costly and require room evacuation. Ozone-based systems may replace ethylene oxide sterilizers and chemical products in the future.
- **Reuse of equipment** – reusable surgical textiles should be tracked to limit number of uses, but are generally more durable (McQuerry *et al.*, 2021). Reusable scrub hats have lower microfibre shed than disposables, which

may reduce infection risks (Markel *et al.*, 2017). Guidelines for laundry of medical linens are available (NHS, 2021b).

- **Lower-impact single-use equipment** – single-use may be necessary for handling infectious materials. Materials that are recycled or plant-based, and of streamlined design are desirable.
- **Hand hygiene guidance** – including hand hygiene stations that use lower-impact dispensing systems and clear signage based on WHO guidelines, alongside training and audit of hand-washing techniques.
- **Monitoring patterns of infection outbreaks** – can identify causal factors or a need for quality improvement within a process.

7.3.5   Buildings, heating and energy

In the UK, energy use accounts for 24% of GHG emissions, and for NHS England, buildings' energy contributes 10% of their carbon footprint. Technological advances may produce efficiencies but rebound increases in consumption are likely; one review observed '*no historical global experience … where energy use falls while GDP continues to grow*' (Brockway *et al.*, 2021). Therefore, rapid decarbonization of energy with demand reduction is needed to sustain our quality of living whilst meeting net zero targets.

Mains electricity is supplied via the UK National Grid, with around 40% currently renewable (wind, solar and hydropower) and the remainder nuclear, natural gas, coal and other fossil fuels. The National Grid is aligned to the government's target of net zero emissions by 2050. Veterinary practices can purchase renewable energy certificates through energy brokers or install on-site technology; grants are available for solar panels, wind turbines and heating systems. Heat pumps and electric boilers are the most practical replacements for gas or oil boilers.

Veterinary clinics are open long hours, with equipment that cannot be turned off, including lighting, and air-cooling for MRI scanners and heat-vulnerable patients. The theatre environment is three to six times more energy-intense than other hospital areas, due to heating, ventilation, air-conditioning, oxygen generators, theatre lighting, active scavenging and forced warm-air devices (MacNeill *et al.*, 2017). Wall/ceiling/floor insulation and LED lighting are priority issues in older and non-purpose-built practices. Further advice on energy efficiency can be found at the Energy Saving Trust or Carbon Trust websites.

NHS England has recently launched a Net Zero Hospital Standard for new hospitals. Sustainability standards for new builds include Building Research Establishment Environmental Assessment Method (BREEAM) and Leadership in Energy and Environmental Design (LEED). Construction carbon emissions can be reduced by 90% by using alternative processes, or materials that are reclaimed, natural or recycled (Sizirici *et al.*, 2021). However, around 85% of a building's life cycle emissions will result from the 'use' phase. Designs can include passive cooling and heat recapture systems, natural lighting and real-time energy monitoring. Building design should promote wellbeing for occupants, by creating green spaces and outlooks (see section 7.4.2), but buildings management systems which improve ventilation in response to occupancy may also improve cognitive performance and health of occupants, although research is conflicting. Wellbeing standards include Fitwel Certification and the WELL Building Standard. Climate adaptation should be considered, for example avoiding construction on floodplains.

Box 7.3. Turn-Off Stickers

In 2020, Linnaeus started distributing plant-based wall stickers. The principles of Nudge Theory mean altering the architecture of an environment to promote a desired choice of behaviour. In this case, stickers placed near switches for lights, computers and air-conditioning 'nudged' people to reduce energy consumption.

To date, around 4000 stickers have been distributed and electricity use across the group has shown absolute reductions despite business growth. The nudge impact may reduce as the stickers become 'wallpaper'; therefore it is important for the nudge to be memorable and a talking point to retain the effect.

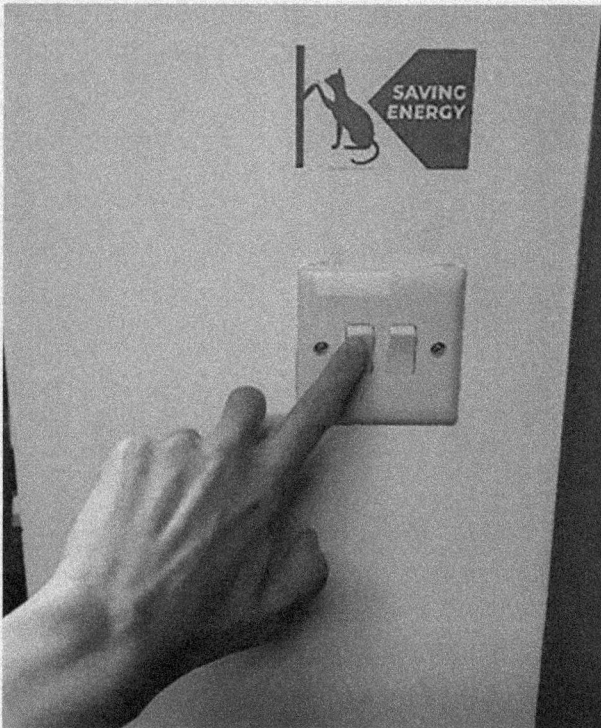

Fig. 7.2. The Linnaeus Paws to Turn Off sticker. (Photograph with permission of Linnaeus, 2022.)

Processes such as end-of-day checklists help to support efficiency. Light turn-off stickers can reduce electricity use by 15% (Rea *et al.*, 1987), but behavioural nudges are less effective and durable than removing unnecessary lighting or automating buildings management systems. See Box 7.3 for an example of a behavioural nudge.

7.3.6   Water

Water-saving measures for veterinary practices include using cistern displacement devices, dual-flush toilets and fixing leaks. Groups such as the Water Footprint Network and Waterwise provide domestic advice on aerating shower heads, greywater use, water-efficient devices and gardening tips. Plant-based diets reduce water consumption; the average water consumption for beef is 15,000 l/kg, compared with 240 l/kg for vegetables (Mekonnen and Hoekstra, 2010). New facilities can have smart-metering and recycling of rainwater and greywater. Co-benefits of water systems include financial savings (reusing rainwater to flush toilets, and water softening reducing inefficiencies due to limescale) and reducing waste (less single-use plastics with use of water distillers or mains-linked water dispensers).

Medical water use is impacted by infection control needs, although high-quality alternatives are becoming available. Alcohol-based surgical hand preparations use 85% less water (Potgieter *et al.*, 2020) and, over their lifecycle, reusable medical textiles reduce water consumption by 250–330% (Overcash, 2012). Steam-cleaners use 90% less water than mop-and-bucket systems, and, depending on the model, can achieve medical bactericidal standards without chemicals.

7.3.7   Transport and active lifestyles

The transport sector is the highest contributor to UK carbon emissions at 27%. For NHS England, 14% of emissions originate from patient and visitor travel, staff commuting and business transport. Further emissions sit within the supply-chain distribution networks.

In the UK, over 60% of journeys under 2 miles are made by vehicle, so there are opportunities for encouraging active travel. Clinics can support cyclists by providing cycle parking, cycle repair equipment, showers and locker rooms. However, many sites are poorly accessible, leaving vehicles as the only option. Driving efficiency starts with planning, which can include grouping ambulatory visits, altering shift patterns to allow lift-sharing, and driver-training courses. Regular maintenance, including optimizing vehicle tyre pressures, improves fuel efficiency. National policies promote electric vehicles, and grants for purchase, charging-point installation, tax exemptions and salary sacrifice schemes are currently available.

A travel policy outlines how a business promotes lower carbon transport and active lifestyles amongst staff and clients. A travel hierarchy can prioritize modes of transport for business purposes, starting with avoiding travel (particularly flights) and prioritizing teleconferencing and teleconsulting. Travel surveys are useful to identify travel preferences and needs. Resources are outlined in Table 7.4.

7.3.8   Digital futures

Veterinary data is stored on paper and electronically, with concerns including storage, accessibility and data privacy. Electronic systems account for 1–2% of global carbon emissions, use rare-earth metals and resources, and create hazardous waste. Whether paper or e-reading is less impactful depends on factors such as use frequency and duration, and storage lifespan. Paper is a renewable resource, with FSC/PEFC certified products, recycled materials and plant-based inks available. Impacts of electronic devices are reduced by purchasing for efficiency, longevity, repair and recyclability. Products with circular design features (e.g. modular smartphones) extend the device lifespan. ICT-specific eco-labels are available. End-of-use options include donating equipment (after data removal) and recycling via approved routes; for both, the end-destination should be transparent.

Table 7.4. Sustainable travel resources.

Type of travel	Organization	Purpose
Active travel	Modeshift	Member organization to increase safe, active and sustainable travel in business, education and community settings
	Sustrans	Resources supporting walking and cycling; manages the National Cycle Network
	CyclingUK	Resources and support for cycling
	Park that bike	An independent transport consultancy supporting cycle parking, surveys and guides
	Bikeability	Cycle training for adults and families
	CycleStreets	Cycle journey planner with fastest and quietest options
	Cycle-to-work scheme	A salary sacrifice scheme for employers to offer to employees
Lower carbon travel	Energy-saving trust	Independent organization providing energy efficiency and clean energy solutions, including lower carbon travel and energy at home
	Traveline	A partnership of transport companies, local authorities and passenger groups providing routes and times, bus, rail, coach and ferry travel in Great Britain

Whilst telemedicine is not new, the pandemic forced the veterinary sector to adopt remote systems to maintain access to care. Purohit *et al.* (2021) found that telemedicine reduced the carbon footprint of medical consultations by 0.70–372 kgCO$_2$e/consultation.

7.4   Sustainability in Our Community

As with many areas of domestic life, pet ownership has environmental impacts, including resource use, carbon emissions and biodiversity losses. The average carbon cost of a dog is 0.8 tonnes of CO$_2$e/year, depending primarily on diet and nationality (Wynes and Nicholas, 2017; Martens *et al.*, 2019). However, studies investigating the carbon 'pawprint' of pet ownership focus on pet food emissions, and rarely include healthcare or lifestyle choices.

Positive sustainability impacts are likely to result from improvement of an owner's mental and physical health, including growing empathy for the natural world (Friedman and Krause-Parello, 2018). Carbon offsetting is gaining popularity, but should be high-quality and accredited by an established agency ensuring additionality, longevity and biodiversity gain. Guidance for net zero-aligned carbon offsetting is available (Allen *et al.*, 2020).

RVNs are well placed to assist owners with lower-impact pet ownership, focusing on preventive care, and diet and lifestyle advice, and to lead within their professional communities. In this section, we examine environmental opportunities for our wider communities.

7.4.1   Pet foods

A pet's diet is likely to form a large part of its ecological footprint, primarily from agricultural practices (Martens *et al.*, 2019). Pet food production is estimated to produce up to 3% of global agriculture's carbon emissions, and in the USA up to 30% of all animal production environmental impacts are attributed to cat and dog diets (Okin, 2017; Alexander *et al.*, 2020).

Consumers have some choice with regard to diets, although pet nutritional needs are complex and vary by species, availability, preference and, in the healthcare setting, pathology. Owners should be guided on suitable diets by veterinary professionals. The Pet Food Manufacturers Association identifies four priorities for sustainability: packaging recyclability; sustainability of ingredients; animal welfare; and other environmental impacts. Research into high-quality options to reduce environmental impacts of pet foods is ongoing. Manufacturers typically mitigate impacts by using renewable electricity, energy efficiency measures, lower-carbon ingredients, deforestation-free supply chains, regenerative agriculture, residual carbon offsetting and using novel nutrients, such as insect protein or algal oils. For instance, insects require less feed and water, have a higher edible weight, and cause up to 100 times lower carbon emissions compared with other livestock species (Cadinu *et al.*, 2020). Finally, food waste currently causes around 8% of global carbon emissions; consumer pet food waste can be targeted by labelling, portion sizing and tackling pet obesity (see Chapter 4, Non-Communicable Diseases and Other Shared Health Risks).

7.4.2   Preventive care, green prescriptions and wildlife

Sustainable healthcare led by veterinary surgeons is often a reactive process, focused on a 'leaner and greener' service. The medical sector prioritizes a preventive approach, with the US 'Choosing Wisely' and UK 'Getting it Right First Time' initiatives guiding on timely and effective investigations and treatment (McGain *et al.*, 2021). RVNs have opportunities to engage owners in focusing on pet wellbeing. This requires excellent teamwork and communication to improve health and wellbeing of pets such that disease states requiring high carbon-cost interventions are avoided, and clients are empowered to manage their animal's condition.

RVNs are frequently involved in managing diseases that may benefit from a preventive approach. These include obesity, nutritional advice (e.g. for diabetic or diet-sensitive animals) and non-pharmacological management of pain, for instance using tools such as Canine Arthritis Management to make lifestyle adaptations (see Chapter 4, Non-Communicable Diseases and Other Shared Health Risks). The RVN may be asked to advise on suitable breeds for an owner; the PDSA's 'Get PetWise' campaign focuses on understanding the 'place, exercise, time and spend' that an animal will need for optimal wellbeing.

Owners may gain mental and physical health benefits from their pets (Martens *et al.*, 2019). For dog owners, there is a 24% reduction in all-cause risk of death, although to protect animal welfare (and in acknowledgement that not all humans enjoy the company of animals) the American Heart Association states that '*pet adoption, rescue, or purchase should not be done for the primary purpose of reducing cardiovascular disease risk*' (Kazi, 2019). Health benefits may result from increased time in Nature. Meeting WHO recommendations for access to green space reduces natural-cause mortality by 2.3% in European cities, which may result from stress alleviation, stimulating social cohesion, supporting physical activity and/or reducing exposure to environmental pollutants, noise and excessive heat (Barboza *et al.*, 2021). Green prescriptions are increasingly used by healthcare providers. Pet owners should be encouraged to avoid impacting ecosystems, including preventing pets from disturbing vulnerable habitats. For example, dog faeces and urine deposited beside paths is linked to over-fertilization of nature reserves with nitrogen and phosphorus (De Frenne *et al.*, 2021). Guidance on avoiding environmental exposure risks from pet parasites and parasiticides is evolving, with a recent position statement from BVA (2021) alongside general guidance from European Scientific Counsel Companion Animal Parasites (ESCCAP).

RVNs also have a role to support biodiversity enhancement, and to communicate those benefits as a trusted voice. Charities such as Plantlife, Butterfly Conservation, Bumblebee Conservation Trust, Wildlife Trust and RSPB have many resources for site-based projects (e.g. bug hotels, pollinator-friendly planting, bird boxes, composting) and citizen-science projects (e.g. Garden Bird Watch, Butterfly Count) for staff to engage with and share. The British Bee Veterinary Association has developed the Bee-Friendly Practice Scheme, encouraging veterinary practices to plant for pollinators. Lastly, the Science-Based Targets Network (2020) has developed resources for businesses to manage their biodiversity impacts, with key performance indicators assessing contribution to water quality, climate change, habitat conservation and pollutant load.

7.4.3   Professional skills, change management and leadership

Whilst One Health is promoted within veterinary teaching programmes, and the Association of American Veterinary Colleges recommended in 2011 that all veterinary students should achieve competency in One Health, the focus is generally on the intersection between animal pathology and public health. Surveys of international veterinary teaching hospitals show *'little evidence that sustainable behaviours are being practiced or showcased despite a strong desire to be more knowledgeable'* (Schiavone *et al.*, 2021). A systematic review of veterinary sustainability literature in 2021 found just three peer-reviewed papers, only one of which focused on small animal care (Koytcheva *et al.*, 2021). Entry-level, degree and postgraduate courses can lead to accreditation by bodies such as the Institute of Environmental Management and Assessment (IEMA) and International Society of Sustainability Professionals. Environmental professionals from all backgrounds may become Chartered Environmentalists.

RVNs typically have multiple roles within their businesses, including clinical and administrative duties, into which sustainability can be integrated. Change management is one of the largest challenges for sustainable healthcare. Whilst there are many models of change management, several components are essential. First, establishing a need for change around a shared vision or value builds engagement. Strong leadership is needed to inspire and empower others. A management position is not necessary to lead, although managers provide the sponsorship or authority to act. Leadership can feel overwhelming but focusing on quick wins can build confidence and buy-in from the team. Secondly, careful planning identifies potential barriers and sets up wins to celebrate. Barriers can include disengaged colleagues, prioritization of other tasks, and a fear of failure. Breaking projects down by setting targets that are specific, measurable, achievable/agreed, relevant/resourced and time-bound (SMART) mean that the outcome, the resource and the time-frame are agreed in advance, leading to a higher chance of avoiding stress or standstill. Addressing existing workloads and eco-anxiety is important; identifying the achievable contribution from the individual to the larger picture is helpful.

Lastly, sustaining the change by careful auditing and communication leads to a culture of sustainability becoming 'business-as-usual'. Communication through multiple channels spreads best practices, but care should be taken to represent work truthfully to avoid claims of 'greenwashing'. In the UK, a Green Claims Code is part of consumer protection law and requires claims to be accurate and clear, supported by credible evidence, to represent the whole story of a product or service without exaggeration, and not to mislead the consumer.

Various tools can be used to assist with change management. These include creating business cases, joining environmental management schemes and following reporting regulations. A business case defines the scope, resource, authority and stakeholders involved in a project, and success can be improved by clear deliverables and careful auditing of performance against pre-agreed indicators. The case for sustainability is strengthened by defining positive outcomes (staff satisfaction, expanding client-base, recruitment and retention, consumer trust, quality of care, financial efficiency, better governance, marketing) and avoidance of negative outcomes (risks to reputation, regulatory compliance and failure to adapt for climate change). The principles of quality improvement initiatives are applicable to sustainability projects, and resources for clinical audits are available through RCVS Knowledge.

Regulatory tools can be used to design and drive energy efficiency measures. Larger UK companies are currently obliged to report GHGs annually. Voluntary reporting is more robust if internationally approved frameworks are followed, such as the Greenhouse Gas Protocol for reporting carbon emissions, the Science-Based Targets Initiative for net zero plans, and the Oxford Principles for carbon neutrality. These help stakeholders to understand your internal processes, although some require specialist support. Lastly, formal environmental management systems and external accreditations will improve the governance of environmental and social issues within a business. Such systems include internationally recognized accreditations such as ISO 14001 or EMAS, or UK-based accreditation schemes such as Investors in the Environment (see Box 7.4).

7.5 Summary

The ecological crises will lead to a redefinition of wealth which recognizes the value of Nature to our society. Change will be hindered by relying on technology, valuing growth without including depreciation of Nature, and a shorter-term outlook. In our clinical work, we must use less, waste carefully, and focus on the value we can add as professionals. Sustainable thinking allows us not only to protect our own communities and way of life, but also to continue to provide high levels of care to the animals that we are responsible for, whether pets, farm animals, or wildlife. As the recent government review into the economics of biodiversity put it: '*our economies, livelihoods and well-being all depend on our most precious asset: Nature*' (Dasgupta, 2021).

Box 7.4. Investors in the Environment

In 2018, Davies Veterinary Specialist became the first veterinary organization to be accredited by Investors in the Environment, a UK-based charity dedicated to supporting businesses reducing their environmental impacts. In 2021, Davies won Investors in the Environment's Natural Environment Champion award for a range of biodiversity projects, including a wildlife camera trap, bee-friendly planting, building bug hotels, installing a barn owl box, wildlife and habitat surveys and a community litter pick.

By 2022, around 100 veterinary organizations were members of the Investors in the Environment scheme, including RCVS, BVA and BVNA. Members work towards accreditation at Bronze, Silver or Green level by appointing Green champions, publishing an environmental policy, measuring use of key resources and setting targets for reduction, calculating carbon footprints, developing waste and travel plans and engaging internal and external stakeholders by communication and project work. Investors in the Environment provides support and online resources, and access to a wider community of non-veterinary businesses.

Within Linnaeus, practice Investors in the Environment leads said that the top business benefits were improving staff morale, marketing, legal compliance and cost-efficiency. For pet owners, environmental accreditations and awards may act as a differentiator when choosing which practice to attend.

7.6   Questions for Further Discussion

1. Which areas do you think could have most impact in your practice: climate change, waste management or resource use?
2. What barriers to implementing sustainable practices do you recognize in your workplace, and what might you gain by overcoming them?
3. Which tool(s) do you think will be most useful to help you reduce your environmental impacts in your day-to-day life?

Acknowledgements

With thanks to Claire Roberts, RVN, for her input on this chapter and Danielle Banks, RVN, for her review of the section on infection control.

References

Alexander, P., Berri, A., Moran, D., Reay, D. and Rounsevell, M.D.A. (2020) The global environmental paw print of pet food. *Global Environmental Change* 65, 102153. doi: 10.1016/j.gloenvcha.2020.102153

Allen, M., Axelsson, K., Caldecott, B., Hale, T., Hepburn, C. *et al.* (2020) *The Oxford Principles for Net Zero Aligned Carbon Offsetting 2020.* University of Oxford, Oxford.

Atwoli, L., Baqui, A.H., Benfield, T., Bosurgi, R., Godlee, F. *et al.* (2021) Call for emergency action to limit global temperature increases, restore biodiversity, and protect health. *Lancet Planetary Health* 5, E660–E662. doi: 10.5546/aap.2022. eng.2

Barboza, E.P., Cirach, M., Khomenko, S., Lungman, T., Mueller, N. *et al.* (2021) Green space and mortality in European cities: a health impact assessment study. *The Lancet Planetary Health* 5, e718–e730.

Bártíková, H., Podlipná, R. and Skálová, L. (2016) Veterinary drugs in the environment and their toxicity to plants. *Chemosphere* 144, 2290–2301. doi: 10.1016/j. chemosphere.2015.10.137

Bennett, M. and Weeks, J. (2021) Current gaps in our knowledge of ectoparasiticides. *Veterinary Record* 188, 200.

Brockway, P.E., Sorrell, S., Semieniuk, G., Heun, M.K. and Court, V. (2021) Energy efficiency and economy-wide rebound effects: a review of the evidence and its implications. *Renewable and Sustainable Energy Reviews* 141, 110781. doi: 10.1016/j.rser.2021.110781

BVA (2011) *Handling veterinary waste. British Veterinary Association.* Available at: https://www.bva.co.uk/resources-support/practice-management/handling-veterinary-waste-guidance-posters (accessed 6 May 2022).

BVA (2021) *BVA, BSAVA and BVZS policy position on responsible use of parasiticides for cats and dogs. British Veterinary Association.* Available at: https://www.bva. co.uk/take-action/our-policies/responsible-use-of-parasiticides-for-cats-and-dogs/ (accessed 6 May 2022).

Cadinu, L.A., Barra, P., Torre, F., Delogu, F. and Madau, F.A. (2020) Insect rearing: potential, challenges, and circularity. *Sustainability* 12(11), 4567. doi: 10.3390/ su12114567

Campbell, M. and Pierce, J.M.T. (2015) Atmospheric science, anaesthesia, and the environment. *BJA Education* 15, 173–179. doi: 10.1093/bjaceaccp/mku033

Dasgupta, P. (2021) *The Economics of Biodiversity: The Dasgupta Review.* HM Treasury, London. Available at: https://www.gov.uk/government/publications/ final-report-the-economics-of-biodiversity-the-dasgupta-review (accessed 6 May 2022).

Defra (2017) *UK Climate Change Risk Assessment 2017.* Department for Environment, Food and Rural Affairs, London. Available at: https://www.gov.uk/government/ publications/uk-climate-change-risk-assessment-2017 (accessed 6 May 2022).

De Frenne, P., Cougnon, M., Janssens, G.P.J. and Vangansbeke, P. (2021) Nutrient fertilization by dogs in peri-urban ecosystems. *Ecological Solutions and Evidence* 3(1), e12128. doi: 10.1002/2688-8319.12128

Deluty S.B., Scott D.M., Waugh S.C., Martin V.K., McCaw K.A. *et al.* (2021) Client choice may provide an economic incentive for veterinary practices to invest in sustainable infrastructure and climate change education. *Frontiers in Veterinary Science* 7, 622199. doi: 10.3389/fvets.2020.622199

Department of Health (2013) *Health Technical Memorandum 07-01: Safe management of healthcare waste.* Available at: https://www.england.nhs.uk/publica-tion/management-and-disposal-of-healthcare-waste-htm-07-01/ (accessed 6 May 2022).

Devlin-Hegedus, J.A., McGain, F., Harris, R.D. and Sherman, J.D. (2022) Action guidance for addressing pollution from inhalational anaesthetics. *Anaesthesia* 77(9) 1023–1029. doi: 10.1111/anae.15785

EC (2018) *Options for a Strategic Approach to Pharmaceuticals in the Environment.* European Commission, Luxembourg. Available at: https://op.europa.eu/en/publication-detail/-/publication/5371e7bd-25db-11e9-8d04-01aa75ed71a1/language-en (accessed 6 May 2022).

Friedman, E. and Krause-Parello, C.A. (2018) Companion animals and human health: benefits, challenges, and the road ahead for human-animal interaction. *Revue Scientifique et Technique* 37, 71–82. doi: 10.20506/rst.37.1.2741

Gatenby, P.A.C. (2011) Modelling the carbon footprint of reflux control. *International Journal of Surgery* 9, 72–74. doi: 10.1016/j.ijsu.2010.09.008

Glidden, C.K., Nova, N., Kain, M.P., Lagerstrom, K.M., Skinner, E.B. *et al.* (2021) Human-mediated impacts on biodiversity and the consequences for zoonotic disease spillover. *Current Biology* 31, R1342–R1361.

Grimmond, T.R., Bright, A., Cadman, J., Dixon, J., Ludditt, S. *et al.* (2021) Before/after intervention study to determine impact on life-cycle carbon footprint of converting from single-use to reusable sharps containers in 40 UK NHS trusts. *BMJ Open* 11, e046200. doi: 10.1136/ bmjopen-2020-046200

Hayes, S. and Froom, S. (2022) The sustainable value of analgesics within the NHS: could adoption of oral pre-operative analgesia reduce the need for IV analgesics? *Anaesthesia* 77(S2), Special Issue: Winter Scientific Meeting 13–14 January 2022, Abstract 83.

HCWH (2018) *Chemicals of Concern to Health and Environment.* Health Care Without Harm. Available at: https://noharm-global.org/documents/chemicals-concern-health-and-environment-0 (accessed 6 May 2022).

HCWH (2019) *Health Care's Climate Footprint.* Health Care Without Harm. Available at: https://noharm-global.org/documents/health-care-climate-footprint-report (accessed 6 May 2022).

HCWH (2020) *Promoting Safer Disinfectants in the Healthcare Sector.* Health Care Without Harm. Available at: https://www.noharm.org/sites/default/files/documents-files/6599/2020-11-25-Promoting-safer-disinfectants-in-the-health-care-sector_WEB.pdf (accessed 6 May 2022).

HCWH (2022a) *Position Paper - Recommendations for Greener Human Medicines.* Health Care Without Harm. Available at: https://noharm-europe.org/documents/position-paper-recommendations-greener-human-medicines (accessed 6 May 2022).

HCWH (2022b) *New Criteria for Sustainable Healthcare Products.* Health Care Without Harm. Available at: https://noharm-europe.org/articles/news/europe/new-criteria-sustainable-healthcare-products (accessed 6 May 2022).

Hu, X., Pierce, J.M.T., Taylor, T. and Morrissey, K. (2021) The carbon footprint of general anaesthetics: a case study in the UK. *Resources, Conservation and Recycling* 167, 105411. doi: 10.1016/j.resconrec.2021.105411

IPBES (2019) *Global Assessment Report on Biodiversity and Ecosystem Services of the Intergovernmental Science-Policy Platform on Biodiversity and Ecosystem.* *IPBES secretariat, Bonn, Germany.* doi:10.5281/zenodo.3831673. Available at: https://www.ipbes.net/global-assessment (accessed 6 May 2022).

IPCC (2022) *Climate Change 2022: Impacts, Adaptation, and Vulnerability. Contribution of Working Group II to the Sixth Assessment Report of the Intergovernmental Panel on Climate Change* (eds Pörtner, H.-O., Roberts, D.C., Tignor, M., Poloczanska, E.S., Mintenbeck, K. *et al.*). Cambridge University Press, Cambridge. Available at: https://www.ipcc.ch/report/sixth-assessment-report-working-group-ii/ (accessed 6 May 2022).

Jeswani, H.K. and Azapagic, A. (2020) Environmental impacts of healthcare and pharmaceutical products: influence of product design and consumer behaviour. *Journal of Cleaner Production* 253, 1–12. doi: https://doi.org/10.1016/j.jclepro.2019.119860

Jones, R.S. and West, E. (2019) Environmental sustainability in veterinary anaesthesia. *Veterinary Anaesthesia and Analgesia* 46, 409–420. doi: 10.1016/j.vaa.2018.12.008

Kazi, D.S. (2019) Who is rescuing whom? *Circulation: Cardiovascular Quality and Outcomes* 12(10), e005887. doi: 10.1161/CIRCOUTCOMES.119.005887

Kennedy, R.R., Hendrickx, J.F.A. and Feldman, J.M. (2019) There are no dragons: low-flow anaesthesia with sevoflurane is safe. *Anaesthesia and Intensive Care* 47, 223–225. doi: 10.1177/0310057X19843304

Kenny, C. and Priyadarshini, A. (2021) Review of current healthcare waste management methods and their effect on global health. *Healthcare* 9, 284. doi: 10.3390/healthcare9030284

Koytcheva, M.K., Sauerwein, L.K., Webb, T.L., Baumgarn, S.A., Skeels, S.A. *et al.* (2021) A systematic review of environmental sustainability in veterinary practice. *Topics in Companion Animal Medicine* 44, 100550.

Lacetera, N. (2018) Impact of climate change on animal health and welfare. *Animal Frontiers* 10, 26–31. doi: 10.1093/af/vfy030

Landrigan, P.J., Fuller, R., Acosta, N.J.R., Adeyi, O., Arnold, R. *et al.* (2018) The Lancet Commission on pollution and health. *Lancet* 391, 462–512. doi: 10.1016/S0140-6736(17)32345-0

Linnaeus (2022) *We go for lower flow*. Available at: https://www.linnaeusgroup.co.uk/about-us/sustainability/wegoforlowerflow (accessed 27 June 2022).

MacNeill, A.J., Lillywhite, R. and Brown, C.J. (2017) The impact of surgery on global climate: a carbon footprinting study of operating theatres in three health systems. *The Lancet Planetary Health* 1, e360–e367.

Mahefarisoa, K.L., Simon Delso, N., Zaninotto, V., Colin, M.E. and Bonmatin, J.M. (2021) The threat of veterinary medicinal products and biocides on pollinators: a One Health perspective. *One Health* 12, 100237. doi: 10.1016/j.onehlt.2021.100237

Markel, T.A., Gormley, T., Greeley, D., Ostojic, J., Wise, A. *et al.* (2017) Hats off: a study of different operating room headgear assessed by environmental quality indicators. *Journal of the American College of Surgeons* 225, 573–581.

Martens, P., Su, B. and Deblomme, S. (2019) The ecological paw print of companion dogs and cats. *BioScience* 69, 467–474. doi: 10.1093/biosci/biz044

McGain, F., Muret, J., Lawson, C. and Sherman, J.D. (2020) Environmental sustainability in anaesthesia and critical care. *British Journal of Anaesthesia* 125, 680–692. doi: 10.1016/j.bja.2020.06.055

McGain, F., Muret, J., Lawson, C. and Sherman, J.D. (2021) Effects of the COVID-19 pandemic on environmental sustainability in anaesthesia. Response to Br J Anaesth 2021;126:e118-e119. *British Journal of Anaesthesia* 126, e119–e122.

McMillan, M. (2021) Sustainable veterinary anaesthesia: single centre audit of oxygen and inhaled anaesthetic consumption and comparisons to a hypothetical model. *Journal of Small Animal Practice* 62, 420–427. doi:10.1111/jsap.13316

McQuerry, M., Easter, E. and Cao, A. (2021) Disposable versus reusable medical gowns: a performance comparison. *American Journal of Infection Control* 49, 563–570. doi: 10.1016/j.ajic.2020.10.013

Mekonnen, M.M. and Hoekstra, A.Y. (2010) *The Green, Blue and Grey Water Footprint of Animals and Animal Products.* Value of Water Research Report Series No. 48. UNESCO-IHE Institute for Water Education. Available at: https://waterfootprint. org/media/downloads/Report-48-WaterFootprint-AnimalProducts-Vol1.pdf (accessed 6 May 2022).

NHS (2021a) *Delivering a net-zero national health service.* Available at: https:// www.england.nhs.uk/greenernhs/wp-content/uploads/sites/51/2020/10/delivering-a-net-zero-national-health-service.pdf (accessed 6 May 2022).

NHS (2021b) *Decontamination of linen for health and social care.* Available at: https://www.england.nhs.uk/publication/decontamination-of-linen-for-health-and-social-care-htm-01-04/ (accessed 6 May 2022).

Okin, G.S. (2017) Environmental impacts of food consumption by dogs and cats. *PLoS ONE* 12(8), e0181301. doi: 10.1371/journal.pone.0181301

Overcash, M. (2012) A comparison of reusable and disposable perioperative textiles: sustainability state-of-the-art. *Anesthesia and Analgesia* 114, 1055–1066. doi: 10.1213/ANE.0b013e31824d9cc3

Parvatker, A.G., Tunceroglu, H., Sherman, J.D., Coish, P., Anastas, P. *et al.* (2019) Cradle-to-gate greenhouse gas emissions for twenty anesthetic active pharmaceutical ingredients based on process scale-up and process design calculations. *ACS Sustainable Chemistry and Engineering* 7, 6580–6591. doi: 10.1021/acssuschemeng.8b05473

Perkins, R., Whitehead, M., Civil, W. and Goulson, D. (2021) Potential role of veterinary flea products in widespread pesticide contamination of English rivers. *Science of the Total Environment* 755, 143560. doi: 10.1016/j.scitotenv.2020.143560

Persson, L., Carney Almroth, B.M., Collins, C.D., Cornell, S., de Wit, C. *et al.* (2022) Outside the safe operating space of the planetary boundary for novel entities. *Environmental Science and Technology* 56, 1510–1521. doi: 10.1021/acs.est.1c04158

Pierce, J.M.T. (2015) *The Anaesthetic Impact Calculator.* Royal College of Anaesthetists. Available at: https://www.rcoa.ac.uk/about-college/strategy-vision/environment-sustainability/anaesthetic-impact-calculator (accessed 6 May 2022).

Ponder, C. and Overcash, M. (2010) Cradle-to-gate life cycle inventory of vancomycin hydrochloride. *Science of the Total Environment* 408, 1331–1337.

Potgieter, M.S.W., Faisal, A., Ikram, A. and Burger, M.C. (2020) Water-wise hand preparation – the true impact of our practice: a controlled before-and-after study. *South African Medical Journal* 110, 291–295. doi: 10.7196/SAMJ.2020. V110I4.14044

Purohit, A., Smith, J. and Hibble, A. (2021) Does telemedicine reduce the carbon footprint of healthcare? A systematic review. *Future Healthcare Journal* 8, e85–e91. doi:10.7861/fhj.2020-0080

RCGP (2022) *Sustainable Development, Climate Change and Green Issues.* Royal College of General Practitioners, London. Available at: https://www.rcgp.org.uk/policy/rcgp-policy-areas/climate-change-sustainable-development-and-health.aspx#gifh (accessed 6 May 2022).

Rea, M.S., Dillon, R.F. and Levy, A.W. (1987) The effectiveness of light switch reminders in reducing light usage. *Lighting Research & Technology* 19, 81–85.

Reynier, T., Berahou, M., Albaladejo, P. and Beloeil, H. *et al.* (2021) Moving towards green anaesthesia: are patient safety and environmentally friendly practices compatible? A focus on single-use devices. *Anaesthesia Critical Care & Pain Medicine* 40(4), 100907. doi: 10.1016/j.accpm.2021.100907

Rizan, C., Bhutta, M.F., Reed, M. and Lillywhite, R. (2021) The carbon footprint of waste streams in a UK hospital. *Journal of Cleaner Production* 286, 125446. doi: 10.1016/j.jclepro.2020.125446/

Rutala, W.A. and Weber, D.J. (2021) Disinfection and sterilization in health care facilities: an overview and current issues. *Infectious Disease Clinics of North America* 35, 575–607. doi: 10.1016/j.idc.2016.04.002

Schiavone, S.C.M., Smith, S.M. and Mazariegos, I. (2021) Environmental sustainability in veterinary medicine: an opportunity for teaching hospitals. *Journal of Veterinary Medical Education* 49, 260–266. doi: 10.3138/jvme-2020-0125

Science Based Targets Network (2020) Biodiversity. Available at: https://science-basedtargetsnetwork.org/earth-systems/biodiversity/ (accessed 6 May 2022).

Sherman, J.D., Thiel, C., MacNeill, A., Eckelman M.J., Dubrow, R. *et al.* (2020) The Green Print: advancement of environmental sustainability in healthcare. *Resources, Conservation and Recycling* 161, 104882. doi: 10.1016/j.resconrec.2020.104882

Sizirici, B., Fseha, Y., Cho, C.S., Yildiz, I. and Byon, Y.J. (2021) A review of carbon footprint reduction in construction industry, from design to operation. *Materials* 14, 6094. doi: org/10.3390/ma14206094

Steffen, W., Richardson, K., Rockström, J., Cornell, S.E., Fetzer, I. *et al.* (2015) Planetary boundaries: guiding human development on a changing planet. *Science* 347, 6223. doi: 10.1126/science.1259855

Stull, J.W., Bjorvik, E., Bub, J., Dvorak, G., Petersen C. *et al.* (2018) AAHA Infection Control, Prevention, and Biosecurity Guidelines. *Journal of the American Animal Hospital Association* 54, 297–326. doi: 10.5326/JAAHA-MS-6903

Thiel, C.L., Woods, N.C. and Bilec, M.M. (2018) Strategies to reduce greenhouse gas emissions from laparoscopic surgery. *American Journal of Public Health* 108, S158–S164. doi: 10.2105/AJPH.2018.304397

UK Government (2022) *Greenhouse Gas Reporting Conversion Factors, 2022*. Department for Business, Energy & Industrial Strategy. Available at: https://www.gov.uk/government/publications/greenhouse-gas-reporting-conversion-factors-2022 (accessed 17 December 2022)

UN (2021) *Sustainable Development. Division for Sustainable Development Goals*. Department of Economic and Social Affairs, United Nations. Available at: https://sdgs.un.org/ (accessed 6 May 2022).

Vozzola, E., Overcash, M. and Griffing, E. (2020) An environmental analysis of reusable and disposable surgical gowns. *AORN Journal* 111, 315–325. doi: 10.1002/aorn.12885

Watts, N., Adger, W.N., Agnolucci, P., Blackstock, J., Byass, P. *et al.* (2015) Health and climate change: policy responses to protect public health. *Lancet* 386, 1861–914. doi: 10.1016/S0140-6736(15)60854-6

West, E. (2021) Reducing the environmental impacts of veterinary anaesthesia. *Veterinary Record* 189, 360–363. doi: 10.1002/vetr.1147

West, E., Woolridge, A. and Ibarrola, P. (2020) How to manage healthcare waste and reduce its environmental impact. *In Practice* 42, 303–308. doi:10.1136/inp.m1678

White, S.M., Shelton, C.L., Gelb, A.W., Lawson, C., McGain, F. *et al.* (2022) Principles of environmentally-sustainable anaesthesia: a global consensus statement from the World Federation of Societies of Anaesthesiologists. *Anaesthesia* 77, 201–212. doi: 10.1111/anae.15598

Whitmee, S., Haines, A., Beyrer, C., Boltz, F., Capon, A.G. *et al.* (2015) Safeguarding human health in the Anthropocene epoch: report of The Rockefeller Foundation–Lancet Commission on planetary health. *Lancet* 386, 1973–2028. doi: 10.1016/S0140-6736(15)60901-1

Wilkinson, J.L., Boxall, A.B.A., Kolpin, D.W., Leung, K.M.Y., Lai, R.W.S. *et al.* (2022) Pharmaceutical pollution of the world's rivers. *Proceedings of the National Academy of Sciences of the USA* 119, e2113947119. doi: 10.1073/pnas.2113947119

WRI (2005) *Millennium Ecosystem Assessment, 2005. Ecosystems and Human Well-being: Biodiversity Synthesis*. World Resources Institute, Washington, DC. Available at: https://www.millenniumassessment.org/en/Reports.html (accessed 6 May 2022).

WWF (2020) *Living Planet Report*. World Wildlife Fund, Washington, DC. Available at: https://www.wwf.org.uk/sites/default/files/2020-09/LPR20_Full_report.pdf (accessed 6 May 2022).

Wynes, S. and Nicholas, K.A. (2017) The climate mitigation gap: education and government recommendations miss the most effective individual actions. *Environmental Research Letters* 12 (07), 4024. doi:10.1088/1748-9326/aa7541

Index

Note: Page numbers in **bold** type refer to **figures** and page numbers in *italic* type refer to *tables*.

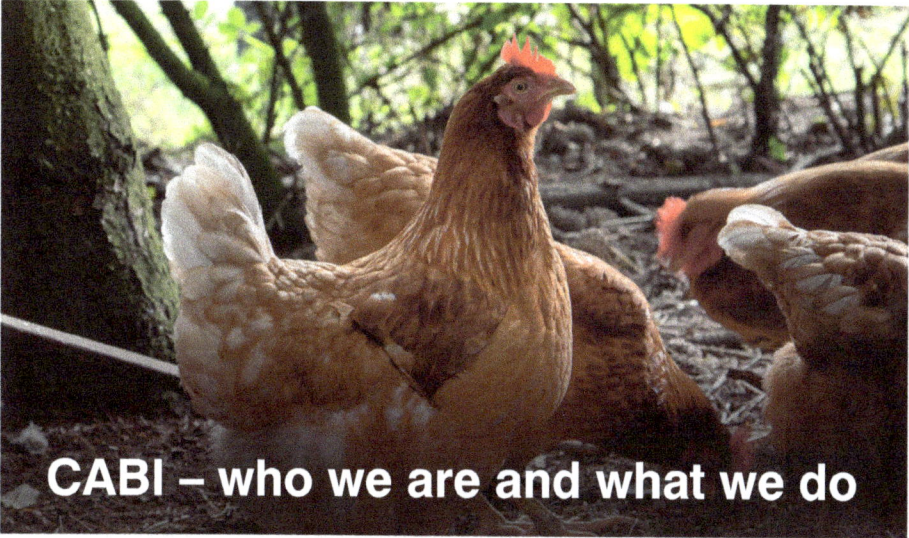

CABI – who we are and what we do

Discover more

To read more about CABI's work, please visit: **www.cabi.org**

Browse our books at: **www.cabi.org/bookshop**,
or explore our online products at: **www.cabi.org/publishing-products**

Interested in writing for CABI? Find our author guidelines here:
www.cabi.org/publishing-products/information-for-authors/